Conversations in

Critical Thinking and Clinical Judgment

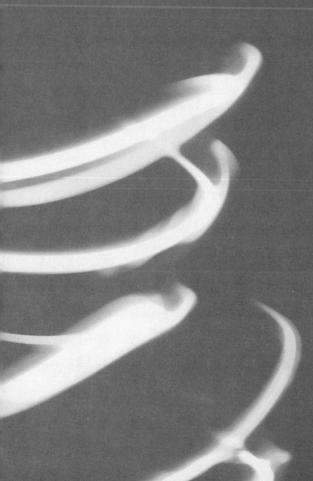

Marilynn Jackson, PhD, MA, RN
Principal
Intuitive Options
Anchorage, AK

Donna D. Ignatavicius, MS, RN
Owner & President
DI Associates, Inc.
Placitas, NM

Bette Case, PhD, BC, RN
Independent Consultant & Partner
Educational Innovations for Healthcare
Chicago, IL

JONES AND BARTLETT PUBLISHERS
Sudbury, Massachusetts
BOSTON   TORONTO   LONDON   SINGAPORE

World Headquarters

Jones and Bartlett Publishers
40 Tall Pine Drive
Sudbury, MA 01776
978-443-5000
info@jbpub.com
www.jbpub.com

Jones and Bartlett Publishers
Canada
6339 Ormindale Way
Mississauga, Ontario L5V 1J2
CANADA

Jones and Bartlett Publishers
International
Barb House, Barb Mews
London W6 7PA
UK

Jones and Bartlett's books and products are available through most bookstores and online booksellers. To contact Jones and Bartlett Publishers directly, call 800-832-0034, fax 978-443-8000, or visit our website, www.jbpub.com.

Substantial discounts on bulk quantities of Jones and Bartlett's publications are available to corporations, professional associations, and other qualified organizations. For details and specific discount information, contact the special sales department at Jones and Bartlett via the above contact information or send an email to specialsales@jbpub.com.

ISBN-13: 978-0-7637-3871-6
ISBN-10: 0-7637-3871-9

6048

Library of Congress Cataloging-in-Publication Data
Conversations in critical thinking and clinical judgment / Marilynn Jackson, Donna D. Ignatavicius, and Bette Case [editors].
      p. ; cm.
   Originally published: Pensacola, FL : Pohl Pub., c2004.
   Includes bibliographical references.
   ISBN 0-7637-3871-9
   1. Nursing—Decision making. 2. Critical thinking. 3. Clinical competence.
   [DNLM: 1. Decision Making. 2. Nursing Process. 3. Judgment. WY 100 C766 2004a] I. Title: Critical thinking and clinical judgment. II. Jackson, Marilynn. III. Ignatavicius, Donna D. IV. Case, Bette.
   RT42.C62 2005
   610.73—dc22
                                2005019013

Production Credits

Acquisitions Editor: Kevin Sullivan
Production Director: Amy Rose
Associate Editor: Amy Sibley
Production Assistant: Alison Meier
Marketing Manager: Emily Ekle
Manufacturing Buyer: Amy Bacus

Composition: Northeast Compositors
Cover Design: Timothy Dziewit
Cover Image: © Photos.com
Printing and Binding: Malloy, Inc.
Cover Printing: Malloy, Inc.

Printed in the United States of America
10 09 08 07 06   10 9 8 7 6 5 4 3 2

Table of Contents

Foreword

Socrates, famous for his ability to gain understanding through questioning, would love *Conversations in Critical Thinking and Clinical Judgment* because it shows the power of asking the right questions. Aristotle would love it because it follows a logical approach and shows that good things happen when bright, committed minds come together. Nurses will love it because it answers many of their burning questions and gives sound, practical advice for how to develop and promote critical thinking skills. These authors have definitely "been there, done that." Now, they tell you how you can do it better.

This book invites you to be a thoughtful participant as some of the most knowledgeable and experienced nurses address some interesting questions. Whether you're involved primarily in practice, education, leadership, quality improvement, or research, you'll find content that is specifically written for you. For example, there's great dialogue on such topics as how emotions affect thinking, how to best foster decision-making skills, and what to do to promote thought-oriented (rather than task-oriented) thinking. There are insights on how to give students and nurses the tools they need to think critically in the context of today's workplace demands, and how to attract, develop, and keep the best critical thinkers on your team. The dynamic question and answer format keeps your interest and helps you move quickly through important content.

These are challenging times that require us to think and learn in new ways. We need creative critical thinkers who are willing to tackle difficult questions together. Yet too often we see leaders who snuff out others' lights to make their own shine. Not so in this book. With Marilynn Jackson at the helm, and Bette Case, Donna Ignatavicius, Jackie McVey, Elizabeth Hand, Krista Meinersmann, and Kathy Missildine contributing, these nurses bring us their best in a unified way. They are to be congratulated on shining a collective spotlight on how to improve thinking and performance.

— Rosalinda Alfaro-LeFevre, MSN, RN
Teaching Smart/Learning Easy
Stuart, FL

Preface

"Advice is like snow; the softer it falls the longer it dwells upon, and the deeper it sinks into the mind."

— Samuel Taylor Coleridge, 1772–1834,
English romantic poet and critic

Don't you love it? A book on critical thinking, and the first page is a "how-to" regarding how to go about making the most of the information. It may be a little presumptuous to assume that a) you will read this intro and b) that you need to in the first place. And as critical thinking is all about validating assumptions, I am proceeding with the idea that you will benefit from the following brief discourse if you are not familiar with the "Conversation" process.

Allow me to briefly explain the background and the intent of this book. Thinking critically, you will remember that keeping an open mind is one of the necessary attributes that allows you to better understand the situation.

First of all, this book is conversational in style and designed to be the kind of experience you would have if you had any one of these consultants nearby and were able to ask those practical, down-to-earth questions that challenge you on a daily basis. A fundamental part of critical thinking, the beauty, and the knowing are in the *question*, as Socrates reminds us.

Each contributor has "been there, done that" and, in several cases, written the book on it as well. The unifying thread is that of critical thinking and clinical judgment, and their experiences are varied, seasoned, tested, and unique. The responses are not theoretical, and while you will find some references, this is not designed to be a formal primer in critical thinking backed by pages of researched references. The research used for the most part is experience, an appreciation for what approaches and strategies work, and what questions inspire, connect, and facilitate the journey toward understanding the elephant.

Oh yes, the elephant. At the risk of being thought "too cute" (remember to keep that open mind) I have adapted the metaphor of the blind men and the elephant. You no doubt remember the story of the four blind men standing at various parts of the elephant and seeking to describe to each other what they "saw"? Each man painted a different picture. Critical thinking is like that: The concept is controversially defined based on where you are standing at the time. Whether you are an educator, manager, seasoned practitioner, or novice nurse on the way to expert, your understanding and approach to critical thinking and clinical judgment will be a bit different. Indeed, even the "experts" have different ideas regarding how to define the concept, as noted in section one.

Much like the blind men, there is no one way to master the elephant. You can read the book at any point and learn a handy tool, gain a new perspective, or validate what you may have also discovered in your role in nursing. The walk around the elephant is designed to have useful information in every chapter for every area of practice, and therefore, is not specifically divided into role application. Managers and educators overlap, and the role of nursing requires many different skills, regardless of your formal position of employment. So, to apply another basic tenet of critical thinking, this book will come at the topic from many angles, and not necessarily in a compartmental or linear fashion.

Time is in short supply for all of us. An index and the table of contents will assist you in pinpointing and going directly to the questions that are most applicable or troublesome to you at the moment. I would not recommend reading the book cover to cover, and in my rather eclectic fashion, I have found that wherever I open the book, I learn a quick lesson that will be useful in some way. I hope you do too—enjoy the journey!

— Marilynn Jackson

About the Editors

Marilynn Jackson, PhD, MA, RN

Principal, Intuitive Options
Anchorage, AK

Completing a doctorate in Business Psychology (2001), Marilynn has shifted her emphasis to intuitive understanding of the personal voice of nursing through reflective practice and the creation of harmony within leadership and work groups. A graduate of the University of Northern Colorado (Greeley, BSN), Marilynn then received her MA in Management and Organizational Behavior from the University of Phoenix. A writer of numerous articles and award-winning books, Marilynn has focused on the concepts of delegation, critical thinking, and outcomes-based care and more recently on the difficulties in the relationships of physicians and nurses. *Clinical Delegation Skills: A Handbook for Nurses*, co-written with Ruth Hansten, was awarded the *AJN* Book of the Year in its first edition, with the third edition released in spring 2004 (Jones and Bartlett Publishers).

Dr. Jackson has recently accepted the position as Executive Administrator of the Alaska State Board of Nursing, and divides her time between Anchorage and the rural setting of Kasilof. Participative sessions and workshops on reflective practice, leadership development, and personal coaching are part of her business, Intuitive Options. Chloe, her resident ray of sunshine (a Golden Retriever), is always at her side, training diligently for a promising future in pet therapy.

Donna D. Ignatavicius, MS, RN

Owner & President, DI Associates, Inc.
Placitas, NM

Nationally recognized as an expert in medical-surgical and gerontological nursing, Donna has a wealth of experiences as a clinical nurse specialist, educator, and nursing administrator for over 30 years. She has taught at the diploma and baccalaureate levels, and most recently in an associate degree program. Currently she provides continuing education and consultation for faculty, staff nurses, managers, and allied health professionals on critical thinking, leadership and management, and gerontology topics through her consulting company, DI Associates, Inc. She has written a number of articles and books, including *Medical-Surgical Nursing: Critical Thinking for Collaborative Care* (4th ed.), *An Introduction to Long Term Care Nursing,* and the *Core Curriculum for Case Management* (with Suzanne Powell). Her most recent article on critical thinking can be found in the January 2001 issue of *Nursing Management.* Donna also has an article entitled "Rheumatoid Arthritis and the Older Adult" in the May/June 2001 issue of *Geriatric Nursing.*

Bette Case, PhD, RN, BC

Independent Consultant & Partner, Educational
Innovations for Healthcare
Chicago, IL

Bette Case practices as an independent consultant to a broad spectrum of healthcare organizations including a travel nurse company, professional schools, professional organizations, hospitals, disease management companies, managed care organizations, a public health department, and providers of continuing nursing education. She assists her clients to achieve their goals using educational, competency management, and quality improvement strategies. Dr. Case is also a partner in Clinical Care Solutions, Inc., which focuses its business on improving medication safety.

She has published on the topics of critical thinking, test construction, competency testing, and career development. She has also written numerous continuing education self-study courses and has prepared competence tests for a variety of nursing specialties. She serves on the editorial board of *The Journal of Continuing Education in Nursing.*

Prior to establishing her consulting practice, Dr. Case held leadership positions in the school of nursing and the nursing department at Michael Reese Hospital and Medical Center in Chicago, IL.

She serves as Membership Chairperson for the National Nursing Staff Development Organization (NNSDO) and was among the first group of nurses to receive certification in Nursing Staff Development and Continuing Education from the American Nurses Association Credentialing Center (ANCC).

Dr. Case earned her BSN at Syracuse University and her MSN and PhD in educational psychology at Loyola University of Chicago, Chicago, IL.

Contributors

Roszlinda Alfaro-LeFevre, MSN, RN
Teaching Smart/Learning Easy
Stuart, FL

Bette Case, PhD, RN, BC
Independent Consultant & Partner
Educational Innovations for Healthcare
Chicago, IL

Elizabeth E. Hand, MS, RN, CCRN
Founder
Hands-On Nursing, PLLC
Broken Arrow, OK

Donna D. Ignatavicius, MS, RN
Owner & President
DI Associates, Inc.
Placitas, NM

Marilynn Jackson, PhD, MA, RN
Principal
Intuitive Options
Kasilof, AK

Jackie McVey, PhD, RN
Assistant Professor
College of Nursing
The University of Texas at Tyler
Tyler, TX

Krista M. Meinersmann, PhD, RN, APN
Clinical Associate Professor
Brydine F. Lewis School of Nursing
College of Health and Human Services
Georgia State University
Atlanta, GA

Kathy Missildine, MSN, RN, CS
Senior Lecturer
The University of Texas at Tyler
Tyler, TX

Section 1:
Walking Around the Elephant: Defining the Characteristics of Critical Thinking

Critical thinking has been enjoying some "positive press" for quite some time now, and you may be wondering what the fervor is all about. More specifically, you may want to know the ins and outs of the definition of this concept, the attitudes, indicators, and models that help to clarify what is meant by this whole process. This section will lay the foundation for thinking critically, exploring many of the confusing aspects from practical angles, and assisting you on your journey around the elephant. Let's get started!

1. **Defining the Concept of Critical Thinking**
   Marilynn Jackson, PhD, MA, RN

2. **Attitudes and Indicators**
   Krista M. Meinersmann, PhD, RN, APN

3. **Assessment and Skills—
   What Makes a Critical Thinker?**
   Marilynn Jackson, PhD, MA, RN

4. **Critical Thinking Models and Their Application**
   Marilynn Jackson, PhD, MA, RN

Chapter 1: Defining the Concept of Critical Thinking

"The limits of my language mean the limits of my world."

—Ludwig Wittgenstein, philosopher

1. Is there one definition for critical thinking that everyone accepts?

Unfortunately (or fortunately, depending on how you look at it!), no. This is frustrating to many who are seeking that "one" perfect summary of the concept. However, the very nature of critical thinking implies that we are open to all aspects, and willing to see issues from a multitude of views, always questioning and challenging the current state. So it seems appropriate that, as critical thinkers, we see many possibilities for descriptors of the process of critical thinking.

There are favorites, and these are often quoted, such as the very simplistic one by Richard Paul from the Center for Critical Thinking in California: "Thinking about your thinking while you are thinking, in order to improve your thinking" (Paul & Heaslip, 1995, p. 42). While this sort of flies in the face of the advice of never defining a word using the word itself, Paul makes a very good point when linking this process to an example: Learning a new skill, and this can be any skill, can be used to illustrate the process to the one who needs further clarification. Consider the task of learning how to perform an intramuscular injection, or learning to drive a car or to ski. While this requires psychomotor proficiency to be developed, it also requires the learner to observe, and think about the process while doing it. Asking "Is this the right location? Is the angle of the needle correct? Do I have the best position?" are evaluative questions that are asked as the skill is developed. This would be similar to thinking critically, that is, asking questions about your thought process: Are these data accurate? What is my attitude about this? Do I have pre-judgments? Do I need more information? These questions are the mark of thinking about your thinking while you are doing so.

2. Are there other definitions that I need to know?

As stated above, there are as many definitions as there are people, and no really "right" or supreme definition. The Internet is a wealth of information, perhaps an overload, but there are several good sites that offer definitions. Community colleges and universities have pages devoted to the topic. You might check out the one for Longview Community College, Lee's Summit, Missouri (**http://www. kcmetro.cc.mo.us/longview/ctac/definitions.htm**).

This beginning page has a compilation of definitions from various faculty and authors and will certainly get you started.

3. Is critical thinking a universal process, or is it limited to a discipline, such as nursing?

Again, we see the struggle of defining critical thinking, and the numerous controversies among scholars, philosophers, and educators. I think it best to leave it to the experts and tend to agree that critical thinking as a concept is a process, or set of skills, that can be applied to any discipline. However, I do believe there are different contextual attributes that make critical thinking specific in interpretation, so that when nurses are speaking of "critical thinking" the application may be somewhat different than what you might encounter in critical thinking in the context of commerce, sales, or educational theory.

Factors that might affect the interpretation and application of critical thinking in a specific discipline include the following:

- Primary goals of the profession
- Moral ground
- Laws and regulations
- Source and precision of knowledge
- Risk/benefit of thinking within the profession
- Relation between thinking and outcomes

4. With all of the varieties of definitions, are there any commonalities that are important to know, no matter what discipline we are discussing?

Similar to a concept analysis, recurring attributes are evident in the majority of definitions regarding critical thinking. There seem to be three repeating and consistent themes, or threads, within all definitions:

1. the importance of a good foundation of knowledge, including formal and informal logic
2. the willingness to ask questions
3. the ability to recognize new answers, even when they are not the norm and not in agreement with pre-existing attitudes

Brookfield (1987), a recognized expert in critical thinking, included the characteristic of "reflective skepticism" in his defined list. This is worth mentioning as a further clarifier of themes 2 and 3 above. Brookfield likened this to continually questioning the status quo, demonstrating an unwillingness to fall into the complacency of doing things the same way "because we always have." Any of us who have been seasoned practitioners in a new job setting have heard this line too many times, and know the frustration of offering a new approach, only to have it soundly rejected. Why would anyone want to consider obtaining daily weights on patients at 8:00 a.m., when we have always had the night shift wake them up at 4:30 a.m.?

5. Critical thinking seems to be the latest "buzz" word. What happened to plain old thinking?

Nothing happened to plain old thinking per se, and it is important to make that clear. When presenting the concept of critical thinking, there are many who will find the idea offensive if it implies that they were not thinking at all in the first place. It will be important to make the distinction, and to employ that age-old tenet of *questioning*, asking the individual what critical thinking involves, and what might be the differences. (The attitudes, behaviors, and indicators of critical thinking are discussed in greater detail in following chapters in Section 1.)

Depending on the setting, I have used a "Socratic dialogue" in which the group is asked the question, "What is the definition of critical thinking?" and then I select someone from the group to begin the discussion while everyone else listens. To assure their attentiveness, I let everyone know I will be calling on the next individual at random, and asking that person to restate what the previous speaker has said, to then seek clarification, and to build on that statement by agreeing or disagreeing with the content. This is a form of "active listening" which assures some degree of focus to override the tendency to be thinking primarily of one's own response, and not fully listening to the statement being shared by the speaker.

6. Why is it important to focus on critical thinking now?

In this era of information overload, it is essential that we take time to consider and reflect upon our actions. With so much knowledge immediately available, it has become apparent that for those who can analyze it and distill the total to that one important small piece that will solve the present problem, it is no longer an easy task. Further, those who can do this and find the needle in the proverbial haystack (now the Internet!) will have economic advantages in the business world as well as other implications for success in the healthcare field.

Another twist is that science has created many new assistive technologies, and while these require skill development, they do not replace critical evaluation of the patient and the surroundings. An infusion pump is a great assistive device, freeing up the nurse from continuously counting drops and adjusting the roller clamp (those of you who are old enough to remember that method!). If the infusion pump is merely set and then ignored, with complete reliance on the alarm system, errors can and do occur. In fact, infusion pumps were cited by the Institute of Medicine (Kohn, Corrigan, & Donaldson, 1999) for a significant increase in medication errors.

7. What is the difference between "regular thinking" and critical thinking?

One would have to be clear about what is meant by "regular thinking," and I would be assuming this to be the quicker, everyday, non-reflective and somewhat reactive processes that we engage in when responses are automatic and not considered. There may be an absence of attention, and a need to "just get it done." The issue at hand may also not be perceived to be important, and as such, a quick response may be believed to be appropriate. This would be what is meant by "regular thinking" (in my opinion, only!).

To make the distinction between the types of thinking, I have often used this definition for critical thinking by Snyder (1993), "The ability to solve problems by making sense of information using creative, intuitive, logical, and analytical mental processes...and the process is continual" (p. 206). This statement includes the idea that critical thinking is a whole-brain process, using both the right side (creative and intuitive) and the left side (logical and analytical), and most importantly, that the process is ongoing. Rather than a linear, end-run approach of regular thinking (i.e., "see the issue/situation/need, take action, and move on"), Snyder's definition is very clear regarding the major differences.

8. Definitions are a good start, but do you have any examples of critical thinking? How do I illustrate what the definitions are describing so that people can understand?

I like to start with fun examples of what critical thinking is *not*, finding that this degree of humor and a light hearted approach can then lead to a more serious, focused discussion on the concept. The key is to start thinking! There are examples everywhere, and I have included a couple of my favorites. You will find others in the appendix on creative approaches.

Some examples are very short and quick, causing the listener to think this is "not quite right," as in:

> I wonder what time they serve the midnight buffet.
>
> What do they do with ice sculptures when they are done?
>
> What is the normal lab value for blood alcohol?

Others come from the clinical setting itself.

When working on an adult med/surg unit as a consultant, I stopped to interview a patient who had just returned from a bronchoscopy. He was settled in bed with his wife at the bedside. The nurse in the room was covering the patient. He was alert, oriented, and noted to his wife and the nurse that he was hungry. Eager to please, and spotting a packet of saltines on the overbed table, the nurse opened them and handed one to the patient. Dutifully, he put the cracker in his mouth and began to chew. It was his wife who saw the difficulty, and she went to get his dentures and a cup of water from the nearby sink. Seems in our haste to serve and to please, we had both forgotten that his gag reflex should be assessed, his NPO status had created a dry mouth, and that the absence of dentures would make chewing the dry cracker very difficult!

9. Those are great examples of what critical thinking is not, so how about an example or two of what it is?

I like to think of the nurse who has just received a new patient assignment. This can occur in any setting, from the clinic to outpatient to home health. No matter where the nurse is, there are a couple of approaches that would indicate the different types of thinking that can occur. Consider these thoughts:

> "I can't take this patient just now—I am already overloaded with work I have not gotten to; I'll never get done on time today...Billy has a softball game, I wonder if I will make it—hope he remembered to take his uniform with him to school...darn, I broke a nail! Sally said the patient has a "difficult family"—great—just what I need! This is one of those days!"

This response indicates both aimless and somewhat disordered thinking, coupled with some of those negative thoughts that only serve to derail what could be effective planning time. There is no doubt that emotion comes into play, and as we see, can interfere with effective reasoning and planning.

Now consider the following thoughts of a critical thinker:

"Hmmm, we're all busy, and it must be my turn to add a patient to my list. If I am going to get out of here on time and be able to see Billy play softball, I will need to change some plans. Better take a few minutes, listen to the report of this patient, and then look at the priorities of what is needed. Since Sally said this patient has a difficult family, I will need to keep an open mind and find out what exactly she means by that. Maybe they just need more information about what is happening."

Rather than the aimless and negative approach of the first response, the critical thinker stays focused, centering mental discipline on what can be controlled and relating that in a somewhat structured consideration of what needs to be done in order to achieve the personal goal of attending the softball game, while also realizing the needs of the patient must be met.

Key ingredients of critical thinking here are emotional control, willingness to take time to plan, and recognition of past experience with difficult families, with the recall that often more information is helpful in reducing that "difficulty" (clinical judgment based on clinical reasoning of past experience and knowledge).

10. What does critical thinking have to do with creativity?

I am tempted to say just about everything! This has been demonstrated through time with nursing, as we have long stated that we are able to provide care despite scarce resources, and to facilitate healing no matter how dire the circumstances. Our creative approaches have often been born of necessity, and the current nursing shortage once again compels us to be ever creative.

I could go on to say that creativity is an innate sense within all of us, and comes to the forefront when circumstances and necessity make it possible, or when the evidence is clear that the standard way of doing something is not going to be possible. New ways are discovered, often through serendipity, and it is then that critical thinking becomes a part of the process, as we seek formalization and a clearer understanding of the applications of the creative idea. For example, consider these creative approaches:

- Sewing a heart pocket on the patient's gown in order to hold the telemetry module instead of letting it drag on the floor or having it drop from the patient's hands. This was one nurse's idea, and now it has been integrated into gowns that are regularly supplied by linen companies.

- Having the resident/patient/rehab client make his/her own bed. This adds a sense of ownership and accomplishment and develops those important skills of daily living.

I'm sure you can think of many more examples and will quickly realize the creative urge is within each of us, seeking expression in a multitude of ways. When we approach a problem critically, and remain open to new and different solutions, we challenge the creative side (right side) of our brains, and the results may be totally unique and yet just what is needed. However, it is risky to be "out of the box," as that generally means challenging the traditional practice and looking at things in new ways. Read more about this in detail in the chapter on barriers.

11. Where does intuition fit into critical thinking?

Benner and colleagues (1999) discussed "clinical grasp" and "clinical forethought" as two components of the process of clinical judgment. Clinical forethought, much like the initial descriptor of intuitive reasoning in the expert practitioner, includes four components:

- Future think (the ability to suspend judgment while planning ahead and preparing for suspected eventualities)
- Clinical forethought about specific diagnoses and injuries
- Anticipation of crises, risks, and vulnerabilities for particular patients
- Seeing the unexpected

I think it is "seeing the unexpected" that is the key ingredient here that relates intuition in one way to critical thinking. One of the primary attitudes of critical thinking behavior is that of suspending judgment and, therefore, remaining open to the possibility that things may not be the same for this patient as for all of the others in this disease category or in similar circumstances. It is that balance point of the expert practitioner who is able to hold the tacit knowledge of past experiences in the background and use that as a stage for evaluating what is different in this current circumstance.

In my doctoral study on intuitive nursing practice, I discovered that there are key similarities and behaviors that nurses employ in terms of "knowing" the patient, and having a degree of predictability of what will happen to the patient in the current set of circumstances. This "knowing," this "gut sense" or immediate apprehension (as Richard Paul reminds us), is an essential trigger point for critical thinking. Without it, I believe we would be missing the essence of nursing practice.

12. Logic and reasoning have been mentioned as components of the critical thinking process, and yet I do not remember learning about logic in the nursing curriculum. How does logic relate to nursing's view of critical thinking?

Logic is a form of thinking that begins with observation and then describes what you do with the data that you collect from that observation. As you make observations and collect data, you begin to see patterns or trends, and form some degree of predictability. For example, a patient returning from surgery is generally groggy, will complain of some pain, and be thirsty. Having taken care of numerous post-surgical patients, when you receive a call from PACU announcing the arrival of another post-surgical patient, you conclude that this patient will act in much the same manner, complaining of operative pain, thirst, and being somewhat sleepy. Moving from a generalized set of conclusions (your pattern of experience with surgical patients) to a prediction of behavior (the patient will be in pain) is an example of deductive reasoning (logical think-ing process).

Likewise, you are working in the labor and delivery room and caring for a young mother-to-be, and her contractions are now less than two minutes apart. She is restless, somewhat anxious, and is fully dilated. You conclude that she is going to deliver this baby very soon, and move her to the delivery room. This is an example of inductive reasoning (no pun intended!), moving from a set of observations to a conclusion that is then verified.

13. I never was very good at logic, and have been told I am not a logical thinker. I am not even sure what it means when someone says, "that's not logical."

Take heart! A foundation of logic can sound formidable, until you realize the components and take it step by step. Logic is really thinking; more specifically, logic is the ability to recognize and analyze the relationships between premises, observations, and conclusions. These tools are part of the foundation of critical thinking, and while you may be unfamiliar with the terms, my guess is that you do them already to some degree. Consider the following syllogism:

All patients with diabetes have erratic blood sugars. (premise)

Joe's blood sugar levels fluctuate. (observation)

Joe has diabetes. (conclusion)

While this may look like a sound argument based on a clear premise, it is the critical thinker who will recognize the assumptions made underlying the premise and challenge the conclusion. Based on your experience, you may know several other reasons that Joe's blood sugar may fluctuate, and this might be a one-time occurrence that is related to his fasting for a religious holiday this past weekend. Or, he may be an athlete and taking steroids, which can also alter the blood sugar levels. In this situation, as a seasoned practitioner and critical thinker, you can say the above example "is not logical."

14. Some people are so passionate about what they are doing, or display strong feelings about their approach to a problem. Where does the emotional component belong in terms of thinking?

Emotions certainly cannot be denied and are often the energy that ignites the spark, or thought, in the first place. Difficulties develop when the emotions take all of the attention, and there is no effort to understand what has created the feeling, where it is coming from, and how it affects the "rational" side of thinking. Damasio (1994) has investigated the effect of emotions on thinking. Goleman (2000) published several books on emotional intelligence, a growing field of study that makes the case for controlling and understanding emotions in order to reason better and make more effective decisions.

Carl Jung did extensive work on the issue of "feeling" as one of the four functions of his typology, and noted that there is a significant difference between emotion and feeling, where feeling is the function that is the basis for "fight or flight" decisions, telling us what is important to us and what is not, and emotion is really the "affect" or the flavoring of the senses. Much further back than Jung, Plato and Socrates also made note of the impact of emotions and thought, beginning the controversy of emotion vs. cognition and what is the importance of each. It is a fascinating study, continuing to play out as we learn more and more about the brain and the "rationality" of emotions. The famous statements "*Know thyself*" (Socrates) and "*I think, therefore I am*" (Descartes) remind us of the very early recognition of the impact of emotions on our ability to reason and to think.

15. I have always considered critical thinking to be a method of problem solving. Some people disagree. Is there more to it?

One of the primary purposes of critical thinking is to achieve understanding. By qualifying points of view and solving problems through questioning, understanding becomes clear. It seems that when we don't question, we fall prey to our own opinions, and often use invalidated assumptions as the basis of our convictions. That's when mistakes can be made, and the trouble often begins, not only in relationships, but also in our effectiveness as practitioners.

Covey (1990) reminds us to "seek first to understand," yet so often we are in too much of a hurry and plunge ahead, taking action that is driven by a quick sense of urgency and perhaps validated only by a sense of "this worked before," or the assurance that we know what is meant. Without seeking clarification, I may make the wrong conclusions when the off-going nurse says to me, "I don't know why this patient is here." Do I conclude that she doesn't know what she is doing, that the patient is misplaced and should be somewhere else, that the patient is too well to be here, or that she just does not care? Is her statement truly a problem, and if so, for whom? It looks like I need more information to better understand her statement. That is part of critical thinking!

While so much of nursing and healthcare delivery is based on problem solving, it is important that we recognize and develop our abilities to identify solutions in the best way possible. This often means suspending judgment and being willing to consider solutions that might be originally thought of as unconventional, and to invest more time in careful reflection in order to determine if the choices made and the actions taken are the best ones.

16. I was told the nursing process was the best way to approach an issue in nursing. How does critical thinking relate to nursing?

Certainly the nursing process, with the step-wise progression of analysis from assessment, defining the problem, taking action in the form of interventions, and then evaluating that action, is a wonderful approach that has been embraced by nursing for a long time. Several studies (Facione, Facione, & Sanchez, 1994; Kataoka-Yahiro & Saylor, 1994; Paul & Heaslip, 1995) have shown in the past that there are distinct parallels and that clinical decision making via the nursing process is related to the process of critical thinking.

I like to think that the nursing process is a discipline-specific approach to problem solving that uses critical thinking elements. My only concern is then emphasizing that the process is continuous, as there are many novice and advanced beginner nurses who believe that the process is an "end-run," and that when the problem is solved, the issue is over. For example, the nurse assesses the patient who complains of pain, an *intervention* is made (often in the form of medication), and the effectiveness of the intervention is then *evaluated*. If the pain is relieved, the issue becomes a task that is crossed off the "to-do" list, only to be repeated the next time the patient complains of pain. Conversely, the critical thinker will continue the process, seeking to determine the cause of the pain, any additional contributing factors such as anxiety, infection, drug interactions, or positioning and continue to work to eliminate or reduce the cycle, leaving the door open for additional attention and creative approaches to pain relief.

17. Staff and literature alike talk about "clinical judgment." Is this any different from critical thinking?

Two nursing authors (Kataoka-Yahiro & Saylor, 1994) have linked the two. They targeted five components:

- specific knowledge base
- experience
- competencies
- attitudes
- standards

Similar to my understanding of the linkage to the nursing process, this connection makes clinical judgment a discipline-specific approach to critical thinking. However, the process is also a bit different, in that clinical judgment involves the formulation and rendering of an *opinion* that will assist the nurse in making decisions about patient care at any given time.

Pesut and Herman (1999) make a somewhat different distinction. They noted that judgment is a process of drawing a conclusion about the distance between the current state and the desired state. For example, in treating a fever, the desired outcome would be a normal temperature. The clinical judgment of a temperature that remains at 102 degrees despite medication would be that there is no match between the desired outcome and the current state; therefore, further actions will be necessary. Their description of judgment outlines three choices:

1) a match between the two states (the fever is gone)
2) a partial match (the fever is reduced)
3) no match (the fever is not gone, and in fact may be higher)

Alfaro-LeFevre (2003) made yet another distinction of clinical judgment, noting that clinical reasoning is used to make nursing decisions about assessment priorities, what issues are significant, and what interventions would accomplish the desired outcome. She suggested nine key questions related to the perspective of clinical judgment:

1. What major outcomes do we expect to see in this particular person, family, or group when the plan of care is terminated?
2. What problems or issues must be addressed to achieve the major outcomes?

3. What are the circumstances? (Who is involved; consider their values, culture, beliefs, and the degree of urgency surrounding the situation.)

4. What knowledge is required?

5. How much room is there for error?

6. How much time do I have?

7. What resources can help me?

8. Whose perspectives must be considered?

9. What's influencing my thinking?

18. What about clinical reasoning? Doesn't that relate to clinical judgment and critical thinking?

Sometimes all of the terms are used in much the same manner, and many believe there is enough similarity that they are the same processes. However, as we have discussed with clinical judgment in the questions above, there is a distinct difference in the process and the outcome of each of these concepts:

- *Critical thinking* is a disciplined process that requires validation of data, including any assumptions that may influence your thoughts, and then careful reflection on the entire process while evaluating the effectiveness of what you have determined is the necessary action to take.

- *Clinical judgment* is the development of opinions in the clinical practice setting, based on experience and knowledge, to guide the decisions you will make regarding the care of the patient. To achieve clinical judgment, you will use *clinical reasoning* in the course of the process, taking clinically specific data regarding specific populations or disease processes and making evaluations regarding their meaning.

I like to consider critical thinking to be the constant overarching component, the method by which we employ clinical reasoning leading to "sound" clinical judgment. If critical thinking were the center of the process, the discipline-specific behavior of clinical reasoning would be the next overlay, and the outer core would be the very specific nursing/clinical judgment (see Figure 1.1). In this way, you can see that critical thinking is used in every way, not just the disciplines of health-care, and that it would be a central component of developing expert practice.

19. Isn't good critical thinking just common sense? I always thought that like common sense, you either have it or you don't.

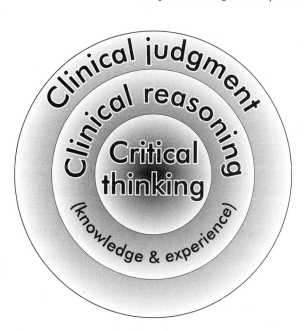

Figure 1.1:   Critical Thinking as the Center of the Process

It's probably true that some of us are better disposed to critical thinking and good judgment than others. And, I suppose that aptitude tests like the *California Critical Thinking Disposition Inventory* (Facione, Facione, & Sanchez, 1994) might sort us out accordingly. But, it's also true that clinical judgment and critical thinking improve with practice and corrective feedback.

One important part of developing clinical judgment and critical thinking is to use the skills on a regular basis—to prevent a sort of cognitive atrophy through disuse. Another important part is the corrective feedback that comes from coaching. Peers, colleagues in other departments, and, depending on the issue, family and friends can all play the role of coach.

Elicit coaching by thinking out loud through the process of clinical judgment or critical thinking. Ask a coach to raise questions about things you may have taken for granted or failed to take into account.

No matter how much we may be like another individual in background and role, we also differ in our personal, educational, and professional experiences. These differences create for each of us a perspective that is unique in some respects. So, seeking the coaching of another can enrich your own perspective by seeing the situation from someone else's vantage point.

The thinking-out-loud technique is especially important in precepting. Usually we think of the preceptor thinking out loud to provide a model for the orientee. However, critical thinking also advances when the preceptor asks the orientee to think out loud in order to offer corrective feedback. This is especially important if something has gone wrong. When you watch a nurse perform a psychomotor skill you can observe each step and offer corrective feedback whenever you observe a misstep. However, with critical thinking and clinical judgment, we usually see only the result—the "how it comes out" as compared with the desired outcome. In order to offer corrective feedback, the preceptor or coach needs to "see" the steps in the thought process.

20. How does critical thinking link reflection to action?

The two components are intertwined, or connected, in the effective practitioner. Much as we discussed the development of the skill of giving an injection, there are two components, or "selves." The active self is the part of an individual's performing a psychomotor behavior, taking action, or demonstrating purposeful motion. The reflective self is that part of the individual watching the action, with the intent of evaluation and analysis in order to improve and to further perfect the activity. The key is to employ both, and to make sure that one does not work without the other. Actions taken without thought and careful reflection are those that do not result in further learning, and they run the risk of becoming mindless tasks of little or no value. However, reflection requires attention, and a willingness to be presently engaged in what one is doing, in order to continue to improve the outcome.

RESOURCES

Alfaro-LeFevre, R. (2003). *Critical thinking in nursing: A practical approach* (3rd ed.). Philadelphia: Saunders.

Benner, P., Hooper-Kyriakidis, P., + Stannard, D. (1999). *Clinical wisdom and interventions in critical care*. Philadelphia: Saunders.

Brookfield, S. (1987). *Developing critical thinkers*. San Francisco: Jossey-Bass.

Cohen, G. (2000). *The creative age*. New York: Avon Books.

Covey, S. (1990). *Principle-centered leadership*. New York: Summit Books.

Damasio, A. (1994). *Descartes' error: Emotion, reason, and the human brain*. New York: Putnam's Sons.

Facione, N. C., Facione, P. A., & Sanchez, C. A. (1994). Critical thinking disposition as a measure of competent clinical judgment. The development of the California Critical Thinking Disposition Inventory. *Journal of Nursing Education, 33*(8), 345–350.

Goleman, D. (2000). *Working with emotional intelligence.* New York: Bantam Books.

Kataoka-Yahiro, M., & Saylor, C. (1994). A critical thinking model for nursing judgment. *Journal of Nursing Education, 33*(8), 351–356.

Kohn, L. T., Corrigan, J. M., & Donaldson, M. S. (Eds.). (1999). *To err is human: Building a safer health system.* Washington, DC: Institute of Medicine, National Academy Press.

Paul, R. W., & Heaslip, P. (1995). Critical thinking and intuitive nursing practice. *Journal of Advanced Nursing, 22,* 40–47.

Pesut, D., & Herman, J. (1999). *Clinical reasoning: The art and science of critical and creative thinking.* Albany, NY: Delmar Publishers.

Snyder, M. (1993). Critical thinking: A foundation for consumer-focused care. *The Journal of Continuing Education in Nursing, 24*(5), 206–210.

Chapter 2: Attitudes and Indicators

"Human beings, by changing the inner attitudes of their minds, can change the outer aspects of their lives."

—William James, 1842–1910, philosopher, psychologist

1. I have heard people talk about someone having "a bad attitude" but I don't really know how they can tell. What are attitudes anyway?

Basically, attitudes are the state of mind or behavior one has about some item, person, or event. Other words that are sometimes used to mean the same thing include:

- standpoint
- outlook
- viewpoint
- feeling
- approach

A quick review of research on attitudes will reveal work done in the social and behavioral sciences as well as nursing on the topic of attitudes (Ajzen, 2001; Batenburg, Small, Lodder, & Melker, 1999; Clark, 1999; Dyson, 1997; Stuppy, Armstrong, & Casals-Ariet, 1998; Vance, 2001). While I like to think of attitudes as the way we look at things in the world around us, more exact definitions can be found in the literature:

- Attitudes are "behavior based on conscious or unconscious mental views developed through cumulative experience" (Thomas, 1997, p. 174).
- An "attitude represents a summary evaluation of a psychological object captured in such attitude dimensions as good-bad, harmful-beneficial, pleasant-unpleasant, and likeable-dislikable" (Ajzen, 2001, p. 28).

To rephrase these definitions, an attitude is a psychological concept that represents the range of feelings someone can have about something, with the range being from negative to positive.

Attitudes develop over time based on previous experiences and embody both conscious and unconscious observations. For example, someone who really enjoys interacting with people and is always very upbeat and positive would be said to have a "good" attitude. On the other hand, someone who is always putting other people down and complaining about things would be said to have a "bad" attitude. So, in this case, we would rather be seen as having a "good" attitude than a "bad" attitude.

Let's say one of your parents is an avid runner. From watching your parent's devotion to training and staying in shape you might develop a positive attitude toward exercise. On the other hand, if you want that same parent to spend time taking you to the park or reading books with you, you might develop negative feelings, a negative attitude, about running because it prevents you from getting what you want.

2. Sometimes I realize I have a particular way of looking at something and I wonder why. How do our attitudes develop?

Well, this is a tricky one to answer. A lot of research resulted in several complex theories on how attitudes develop and how they may change over time or from context to context. In general, attitudes seem to develop out of our experiences with the world. Initially they may be based on the way we are socialized as children. Socialization occurs first in our homes from our interactions with our family. We learn from how we are treated and how we see others around us treated.

To simplify these complex theories, consider the following progressive list:

- Attitude development starts in childhood based on how we are socialized at home.
- Attitudes may be reinforced or challenged when we enter the educational system.
- Interactions with mentors, peers, employers, and teachers may alter initial attitudes.
- Experiences in the world may cause us to think critically about and question our attitudes.

3. If our attitudes occur without our really realizing it, why study or even think about attitudes?

It is important to recognize how you think or feel about things that occur in the world around you. If you just live your life without ever questioning your attitudes, without thinking critically about your attitudes, then it seems to me that you are living life on automatic pilot and not really living life to your fullest potential.

When I traveled to Haiti with a group of students to provide healthcare to Haitians who had little or no access to such care, I had an opportunity to challenge the conventional attitude that money and possessions bring happiness.

The people we met were friendly and welcoming; they had positive attitudes yet they lived in a state of poverty unlike any I had seen before. People were living in abject poverty without running water or plumbing, in cramped housing with dirt floors, and minimal to no furniture. The students and I had to take a critical look at what attitudes we held about money and happiness as we viewed the lives of the people for whom we cared.

4. I have never really focused on why I think and feel the way I do about things. How can we recognize our own attitudes?

Let's try looking at an example. You are in a mall and you find a wallet lying on the ground. At first you just start to walk away but then you turn and pick the wallet up and take it to the mall office. To understand the attitudes that influenced your behavior you might want to answer the following questions: Why did I do this? What influenced my actions? Why didn't I keep the wallet or just leave it there? Why did I hesitate at first? The answers to these questions will help you get to the bottom of your behavior, to the attitude that influenced your behavior. Your answers might be that you were afraid of being accused of stealing the wallet or of getting involved in something that did not concern you; therefore, you started to walk away. But then you realized that the right thing to do would be to pick up the wallet and give it to the proper authority. This was the right thing to do because the person who lost the wallet had the right to have it returned. After answering these questions, you might decide that the attitude that influenced your behavior was that being an honest and ethical person was more important than avoiding involvement.

Steps to learning to recognize your attitudes:

- Develop the ability to question yourself.
- Pick a situation where you acted a certain way and don't know why.
- Think critically about your behavior in the situation.
- Make a list of what influenced your actions/feelings.
- Be open and honest with yourself.
- Practice the above steps with a variety of situations.

The same type of reflective analysis can be applied to patient care. Suppose you are a nursing student and you have been assigned to care for a homeless individual. Your first reaction might be very negative. As you reflect critically on this reaction you may realize that you have an attitude that all folks should work for a living. This may come from a parental message regarding the need to earn what you have. You assume that the patient does not work or he/she would not be homeless. So your negative attitude toward homelessness is making you have a negative reaction to this patient assignment. Being aware of your attitude and what motivates it is the first step in being able to give this individual appropriate care.

5. Sometimes when I try to decide what I think about a particular situation I cannot figure it out. Is there a strategy to help with this reflection?

I think we can know what our attitudes are, if we really want to figure them out. The most important thing involved in discovering what your attitudes are is being willing to take the risk to be totally honest with yourself, and to overcome the fear of being vulnerable. Journaling can help with this; it is a great habit to develop, and there are even computer programs to assist with the process. If you don't work that much on a computer, there are wonderful bound books in any stationery store.

How to identify your attitudes:

- Risk being open and honest with yourself.
- Keep a reflective journal of your thoughts, feelings, and actions.
- Think critically about your behavior and what influenced the choices you made.

6. So now that I know how to recognize my attitudes, how can I figure out how they influence my choices/actions?

Let's look at this in a little different manner. Instead of looking at what you think influences your behavior in a situation, look at *why* you think these things influenced your behavior. Consider finding a wallet in the mall. Your attitude of being an honest and ethical person compels you to turn the wallet into store security. Couldn't you have just opened the wallet and seen if there was any identifying information in the wallet that would help you to return it yourself? That would still reflect your attitude that being honest and ethical is important, wouldn't it? But now you realize that the idea of solving the problem that way is causing you to feel anxious. On further honest appraisal, you realize that you have a negative attitude toward interacting with strangers, which made this option much less desirable. The further analysis has helped you to realize that a variety of attitudes influenced the choice you made in this situation. So again, critical and open appraisal of your behavior and the attitudes underlying them has helped you see how these attitudes influence your choices/actions.

7. I have realized I don't like some of my attitudes. Is it possible to change our attitudes?

Changing attitudes typically involves critical thinking. An open mind and the ability to look at other options and to reflect on why you are doing what you are currently doing are all part of the process. For example, I realized a while back that I really was not getting enough exercise. Now I had been a runner for over 15 years off and on, more on than off, but for some reason I was currently not getting any regular exercise. I reflected critically on this for a while and realized the change had happened when I developed problems with one of my feet. I had spent about a year working that out but had not started exercising again. Time had gotten in the way, and I had sacrificed the good feelings I had when exercising and had developed the attitude of not having enough time, so why bother? Challenging myself to look at what was more important, I set a goal of trying to walk at lunch each day while at work and got some friends to join in. Before long I was walking at least one mile a day five to seven days a week. I felt great. My attitude has become one of taking better care of myself as a top priority.

Steps to changing attitudes:

- Recognize the attitude you want to change.
- Determine why you have the attitude and what need it serves.
- Decide what new attitude you want to adopt.
- Set gradual goals for attaining the new attitude.
- As each goal is met, congratulate yourself and move on to next goal.
- Over time the new attitude will become ingrained in your behavior.

8. Besides not liking them, why might I want to change my attitudes? What is there to gain from changing them?

As we have already discussed, many of our attitudes develop without our conscious thought, almost like osmosis. Think about yourself as a giant sponge that soaks up attitudes from the environment much like the sponge soaks up liquids. Now the thing is that many of the attitudes we soak up come from commercial sources such as television and radio. The folks who are putting the attitudes out there for you to soak up have something to gain from your taking on the attitudes they are portraying. If we do not take the time to reflect critically on our attitudes we are in many ways living life in the dark and behaving in ways that someone else desires. After critical reflection it may be that we decide we like the attitudes we have developed over time and do not want to change. That is fine because you have made the conscious choice to keep the attitudes.

Critical reflection may also allow you to recognize attitudes that do not serve you well or are even detrimental. For example, it is not uncommon for young women to believe that they are overweight when they weigh less for their height than recommended. They have been bombarded with visual and audio messages that thin is in and fat is out. Without thinking critically about these messages, they have taken on the attitude that is it good to be thin and bad to be anything other than thin. These unconsciously acquired attitudes can lead to health problems and, taken to the extreme, death. So in this case, reflecting critically on your attitudes and working to change them could be life saving.

9. **We often hear that it is important to have appropriate behavior in certain situations. Is the same true for attitudes, and, if so, what are appropriate attitudes?**

I think to a certain degree we each have the responsibility and obligation to decide for ourselves what the appropriate attitudes are for us to have. That said, let me add that there are times and places when appropriate attitudes are determined by the situation and setting. For example, certain career choices carry with them both explicit and implicit expectations about the appropriate attitude for someone in that career to have. Teachers are expected to come to school with a positive attitude about their students and a willingness to help them learn. Firefighters are expected to be willing to put their lives at risk to help others; in other words, to have an attitude of selflessness in the face of danger.

I have worked in a variety of institutions and have often found that there were expectations about the attitudes I should portray. In one such institution there was the expectation that the employees would always portray a very positive, can-do attitude with each other and with outsiders. The same is true for nursing, and in fact, most nurse practice acts discuss the expected behaviors in caring for patients in a moral and just manner.

10. **Many times we are judged by our behavior but often our behavior is not a true indication of our true self. What would be an ideal way to display our attitudes?**

Many times I am not really aware of or conscious of my behavior. I am not thinking critically about what my behavior is communicating to others, of what attitudes I am displaying by my behavior. I recently had the unpleasant experience of having this pointed out to me rather explicitly. I was part of a team evaluating a healthcare institution. After the evaluation visit was over, I was confronted with the information that it was believed by some that I had a very negative attitude toward the institution and had negatively influenced the evaluation. I was stunned by this revelation. I thought the visit had gone very well and felt very positive about the institution. I really had to stop and do a lot of critical thinking about the visit. I eventually realized that my behavior was a reflection of a variety of things that had transpired during the visit which were not related to how I felt about the institution. Evidently my external behavior did not match my true attitude about the institution. This has made me pay much closer attention to what my body language is saying to others. I consider myself to have a very positive overall attitude about life and I want my behavior to reflect that attitude.

I would say that the best way to display your basic attitudes is to reflect critically on how your behavior is interpreted by others. Ask your friends, employer, teachers, and family to tell you what attitudes they think your behavior portrays. Then figure out if what they say fits with the attitudes you want to convey to the world. If they fit, then carry on with what you are doing. It is obviously working. But if you are conveying some attitude that is not a true reflection of yourself, then it is time for some critical thinking and behavior or attitude change.

11. As a nurse I need to be aware of the impact of things on my patients. How will being a critical thinker influence my attitudes about patient care?

As we have seen, our behavior is often influenced by our attitudes, whether we are aware of them or not. As a nurse it is important to put the patient's needs and safety first. Additionally, it is important to be considered a team player, one who works with the group to accomplish the goals of safe, effective, and quality patient care. Being able to do these things involves adopting a variety of positive, professional attitudes. So being able to think critically about the attitudes you have and determine if they will impede or enhance your effectiveness as a nurse is very important.

12. Why is it important to learn to be a critical thinker in today's diverse work environment?

When I entered nursing over 25 years ago, most of the people I worked with and cared for were Caucasian or African American. Today, the patient care environment is much different. The nurses providing care are composed of a wider variety of races and ethnic origins. The patient population has changed even more and has become extremely diverse. Often you will find yourself caring for someone whose native language is not English and who speaks little or no English. I have found myself working with a wide variety of interpreters from taxi drivers to the eight-year-old boy who lived next door.

This incredible diversity demands the ability to be a critical thinker.

Basic nursing skills often depend on your ability to communicate with the patient and gain cooperation. If you cannot speak the patient's language you have to think critically about other ways to communicate. I worked with a male nursing assistant years ago in a rural hospital that also served as the public health hospital for ships traveling to a local port. I remember one patient from Turkey who was brought by helicopter to the emergency room and admitted. I needed a urine specimen from him for a lab test. The male assistant went in and tried repeatedly to explain to the man what was needed. In desperation and after some on-the-spot critical thinking, he got a second urine specimen container and demonstrated to the patient exactly what he needed the patient to do! I was amazed at the ingenuity he displayed in accomplishing his assigned task. This is the kind of critical thinking that will be needed to meet the needs of the increasingly diverse patient population.

13. How can critical thinking change the way we look at our attitudes?

Attitude formation or development is often a totally unconscious process. As we develop the ability to think critically we also develop the ability to participate in self-reflection. It is only by critical thinking and reflecting on what we think and believe and how we behave in the world that we can come to know what our attitudes about life truly are. Learning to think critically about our attitudes allows us to identify them and then decide if we want to change them or keep them.

For example, many nurses have negative attitudes about patients who do not follow their recommendations about health promotion activities. These patients are considered noncompliant. Over time I have used critical thinking and reflection in regard to patients who are considered noncompliant. I have realized that the term noncompliant perpetuates a negative attitude toward patients. This is not an attitude that I want to portray to anyone: patients, students, nurses, or other members of the healthcare team. After much critical thinking and reflection, I have decided to look at these patients as exercising their freedom of choice and their choice is not always what the healthcare team recommends. Reframing this situation has helped me change my attitude about these patients to one that is more positive and is based on the recognition of their right to make their own choices. In this case, critical thinking definitely influenced my attitudes in a positive manner.

So, in way of review, critical thinking allows for:

- Reflection on own behavior
- Identification of underlying attitudes
- Examination of the relationship between attitudes and behavior
- Readjustment of attitudes if desired

14. How can examining my attitudes about various topics and issues improve my ability to be a critical thinker?

Critical thinking, like any new skill, takes practice. Using critical thinking to examine your attitudes will help you become more adept at using critical thinking. This is much like learning to give medications. When we first learned this skill we had to state the five rights out loud for the nursing instructors. With repetition these essential steps in medication administration became entrenched in our brains. So, too, with critical thinking. Repeated practice in critical thinking about our attitudes regarding a variety of topics and issues will help us develop better critical thinking skills.

15. Why can we easily encourage others to change or adjust their attitudes but have difficulty changing our own?

I think the answer to this question lies in part to the fact that we can easily observe other people's behaviors. In so doing we are able to make a determination about what their behavior reveals about their attitudes in general. Then we can confront them with our observations. It is up to them to do the work to determine if our observations and judgments about their attitudes are accurate or not. Encouraging others to change or adjust their attitudes is also easier because we can maintain the status quo in our own lives. When we are working on our own attitudes we have to be willing to be open and honest with ourselves. We need to be willing to engage in a process of change. Sometimes this may involve critical thinking regarding issues that cause us discomfort and even emotional pain. But when we confront a peer we can cut to the chase and then walk away. However, it is important to realize that the individual you are critiquing will suffer the same difficulties in changing attitudes as you do. Most important, the person will need to evaluate your input and determine if it is valid.

16. How can we help our peers recognize their attitudes and how these affect their interactions with others?

I think the way we can best help peers is to find a way to be a mirror for them that reflects their attitudes back to them without causing discomfort. This is not an easy thing to do, and it involves confrontation that comes from a win-win point of view rather than a win-lose point of view. You might start by identifying the attitudes you think your peer holds that are nonproductive or even detrimental to interactions with patients, peers, other members of the healthcare team, or family. Then pick the one that is in most need of adjustment as the focus of your work with the peer. Once you have determined what you will focus on, share your observations with your peer. This can best be done by using statements that avoid blame and are not accusatory.

To help peers change attitudes:

- Be a mirror for their behavior.
- Use a win-win approach.
- Avoid blame.
- Be supportive and positive.

For example, you have noticed that the individual is very short-tempered with older patients who require assistance with their activities of daily living. You might start by saying something like, "I noticed that Mrs. Smith needed a lot of extra help with her breakfast tray this morning. Sometimes I find this very difficult to handle and I get frustrated and angry with her. But I have found that spending the extra time with her upfront and conveying a positive attitude about helping her, reduces the number of times I have to return to her room during the next hours. Do you think a similar approach might work for you?" In this manner you have opened the door for dialogue and not made your peer feel put down or criticized. Usually, this is all it takes to get the dialogue going and in most cases the peer already knows he/she has an attitude that needs changing, but just needs some help getting the process started.

17. How can we help peers to recognize that it is important to think critically about their attitudes?

I think this is a time when going to the literature might be helpful. Find articles that have studied nurses' attitudes and patient care. If there are any studies that directly apply to your practice area then share them with your peers. If there are none that seem to directly apply try to select a few that are broad enough to be relevant to your area of practice. You can share them by circulating them among the staff and then set a day for a group lunch to discuss the articles. At this time you can portray a positive and enthusiastic attitude toward thinking critically about and challenging your own attitudes. In this manner you serve as a role model for your peers. If you find you cannot get your peers to read the circulated article, volunteer to do a presentation for the group or to make a poster to put in the break room that summarizes the article. In all interactions with your peers try to reflect a positive and enthusiastic attitude. This will be contagious and will encourage others to be more positive and enthusiastic also.

18. Are there ideal attitudes that all nurses should display? Why or why not?

From the earlier discussion we can see that there are indeed ideal attitudes that nurses should display. They are often referred to as professional attitudes or characteristics. An excellent overview of some of the ideal attitudes nurses should display is offered by Alfaro-LeFevre (2003). She identified 17 ideal attitudes of critical thinkers in the following list, all of which apply to nurses, and are similar to the attitudes discussed in Chapters 1 and 3. While employers cannot really prescribe attitudes, you will typically find similar character statements in the values and mission statements of healthy organizations.

Ideal Attitudes for Critical Thinkers

Active thinker	Honest
Fair-minded	Proactive
Persistent	Organized and systematic
Good communicator	Flexible
Open-minded	Realistic
Empathetic	Cognizant of rules of logic
Independent thinker	Team player
Curious and insightful	Humble
Creative and committed to excellence	

The attitudes delineated in the preceding list are important for all nurses to adopt because they are essential to doing nursing work competently and effectively. When providing patient care, nurses must be able to work with a group of people, so being a team player and having good communication skills are essential attitudes. The current healthcare delivery system requires that nurses take care of a greater number of patients who are often very sick. To do this effectively nurses need to be organized, proactive, and systematic in their provision of care. At the same time they need to be prepared for the unexpected which requires them to be active thinkers and to be flexible.

19. What would be the benefit of having a standard of ideal attitudes for all nurses?

In the previous question we looked at ideal attitudes whereas in this question we are looking at standardized attitudes. Standardized attitudes are more formal than ideal attitudes and are usually developed by nursing practice organizations such as the American Nurses Association (ANA). The ANA has developed standards of practice for nursing in general as well as for some nursing specialty areas. In addition many specialty organizations have also developed discipline-specific standards of practice. In June 2001 the ANA House of Delegates approved a Code of Ethics for Nurses that lists nine statements regarding the appropriate ethical behavior that all nurses should portray (ANA, 2001). Many of the behaviors listed in the Code describe appropriate attitudes that nurses should portray.

Using standardized lists of ideal attitudes to guide nursing practice helps provide consistency in care across educational levels and practice areas. A common set of ideals also helps nursing present a unified voice to the public when it comes to issues that are important to nursing and nursing care. Additionally, using standardized attitudes to guide patient care will benefit patients by ensuring that they all receive appropriate care.

20. How could we encourage others to espouse appropriate attitudes?

I think there are really three simple steps to accomplish this:

- Act as a role model in all that you do.
- Treat all members of the team with respect.
- Provide educational programs on the topic.

21. If we think critically about our attitudes, what unique possibilities might emerge?

I think the possibilities are endless. If we let history lead the way we can see how critical thinking and reflection by nurses in the past has moved the discipline from being handmaidens to physicians to being collaborators in patient care. We have cast aside an attitude of servitude and taken up an attitude of partnership and collaboration. Who can tell what possibilities might emerge in the future if nurses continue to use critical thinking to examine our attitudes about patient care and life in general?

The push to provide evidence-based practice is one area of nursing where nurses' attitudes may be putting up walls that are counterproductive. Nurses often indicate an abhorrence of nursing research. Yet if nursing as a discipline is to survive nurses must prove that our care makes a difference. One way to do that is to use evidence-based practice. So critical thinking about our attitude toward nursing research may allow us to overcome our negative attitude and fully embrace the concept of evidence-based care. This would be a giant leap forward in proving the importance of nursing care to patient outcome and could ensure the survival of the discipline for years to come.

As I said at the start—I think the possibilities are endless. Let your mind go and think critically about where you would like to see nursing. Then reflect on what is holding nursing back or failing to encourage its growth, what attitude is getting in the way? Once you have figured that out you are well on your way to helping the profession move into new ventures for the future. Keep that critical thinking cap handy as we move into the future. We will need it to meet the challenges ahead.

RESOURCES

Ajzen, I. (2001). Nature and operation of attitudes. *Annual Review of Psychology, 52*, 27–58.

Alfaro-LeFevre, R. (2003). *Critical thinking in nursing: A practical approach* (3rd ed.). Philadelphia: Saunders.

American Nurses Association. *Code of ethics for nurses—provisions*. Retrieved May 23, 2002, from **http://www.nursingworld.org/ethics/chcode.htm**

Batenburg, V., Smal, J. A., Lodder, A., & de Melker, R. A. (1999). Are professional attitudes related to gender and medical specialty? *Medical Education, 33*, 489–492.

Clark, A. (1999). Changing attitudes through persuasive communication. *Nursing Standard, 13*(30), 45–47.

Dyson, J. (1997). Research: Promoting positive attitudes through education. *Journal of Advanced Nursing, 26*, 608–612.

Stuppy, D. J., Armstrong, M. L., & Casals-Ariet, C. (1998). Attitudes of health care providers and students towards tattooed people. *Journal of Advanced Nursing, 27*, 1165–1170.

Thomas, C. L. (Ed.). (1997). Taber's cyclopedic medical dictionary (18th ed.). Philadelphia: F. A. Davis.

Vance, D. K. (2001). Nurses' attitudes toward spirituality and patient care. *Medical Surgical Nursing, 10*, 264–268.

Chapter 3: Assessment and Skills—What Makes a Critical Thinker?

"Even as water carves monuments of stone, so do our thoughts shape our character."

—Hugh B. Brown, Canadian-American religious leader

1. How do I know if I can think critically?

I am reminded of Tom Peters' famous response about quality, "I know it when I see it." Critical thinking seems to be much the same way, and although we have established some behaviors and criteria, along with a skill set, we are still not in complete agreement regarding exactly what critical thinking is. Consider its relationship to intelligence and problem solving, for example. You will often hear, "He/she is pretty smart, but lacks common sense," but you will seldom hear, "He/she is smart, but not a good critical thinker."

How will you know if you are a critical thinker? Ask others to give you feedback on your decisions; share thinking out loud with colleagues and compare with their approaches; spend time reflecting on your decisions and the results you have achieved. Evaluate with others whether you are open minded and willing to look at other views, or whether you are too rigid in your approach, and married to your habits. Critical thinking is a work in progress, a continual process to be engaged in. By virtue of asking the question, you are open to information about where you are in the development of the necessary skills. The following questions should help give you even more direction.

2. I am often told I do things the "old-fashioned way." I assume this is not a positive comment, as the complaint is usually made that I take too long and am a bit stubborn. Are these approaches different from critical thinking?

Sounds like you are being described as a traditional thinker. While it is not a good idea to categorize, much can be learned by looking at families of characteristics to self-assess and then to determine what differences you would like to make in your style. While the "traditional thinker" column in Table 1 seems rather negative, challenge yourself by asking, are there times when a "traditional" approach would make sense?

TABLE 3.1 What Is Your Thinking Style?

The traditional thinker…	The critical thinker…
• Preserves the status quo: "This is how we always do it."	• Questions the questions; asks "Why?"
• Accepts the norm and the daily routine	• Is open to possibilities
• Treats each patient and event in isolation	• Views each patient and event as part of a larger group
• Doesn't make connections between patients and events or clinical knowledge	• Looks for patterns and trends
• Has a limited scope and vision	• Has a wide scope and vision
• Accepts the obvious without questioning or exploring other options	• Uses intuition and follows hunches
• Solves problems in isolation—focus is only on fixing the current problem by oneself	• Seeks out experienced peers to use as sounding boards when solving problems

3. I heard somewhere that critical thinking was a basic trait, and you were either born with it or not, and there was little that could be done. Can critical thinking be developed?

This question has challenged many, as there seems to be an indication that some people are better thinkers, make better decisions, and see things more readily than others. However, what is the reason that they can do so? Is it a product of their genes, their education, their environment, or their upbringing? When we consider the skills and aptitudes that are now part of the consensus of what defines critical thinking, it would seem to me that these are skills that can be developed and improved upon with time, practice, and focus.

Thinking critically and being open-minded, I would have to say that anyone (who is not mentally impaired) can improve the ability to reason and to understand, and to better problem solve through more effective communication skills and an increased understanding of self. I know from personal experience that the journey from high school through the attainment of advanced degrees has increased my knowledge base, formalized my communication skills, and helped me to be more systematic in my approach to problems. Has it made me a better critical thinker? Yes, as I have improved many skills through the years, and I am more confident in my decisions and choices now.

4. What are these basic skills that are a part of critical thinking?

A Delphi research study conducted in 1989 by the American Philosophical Association (APA) resulted in the creation of both a consensus definition of critical thinking and a list of both cognitive skills and personal attributes to describe the critical thinker. The six cognitive skills (adapted from Facione, 1996) are described in Table 3.2. These skills include:

- Interpretation: categorizing, clarifying, and decoding
- Analysis: ideas, identifying and analyzing arguments
- Evaluation: assessment of claims and arguments
- Inference: challenging evidence, alternatives, and conclusions
- Explanation: results, procedures, and arguments in terms of validity and justification
- Self-regulation: assessment and correction

5. If there is a list of general skills, is there something that has been developed that is specific to nursing?

Continuing with the premise that critical thinking is a universal process that has context-specific influences, it is reasonable to expect that there would be skills specific to nursing. And so, another Delphi study was conducted among expert nurses in nine countries, during the years 1995–1998. The article makes interesting reading for the description of the process and a summary of the conclusions reached by this panel of 55 nurses (Scheffer & Rubenfeld, 2000).

Since we are looking at a specific context, it is important to note the differences between the general skills and the ones determined by the nursing-specific study. Table 3.2 lists the results of each study. Nursing agrees with several of the general skills, adding the following skills:

- Applying standards: judging according to personal, professional, and social rules
- Predicting: envisioning a plan and the consequences
- Transforming knowledge: changing the condition, nature, form, and function of concepts among context

6. Lists of skills are helpful, but how does this translate in the real world? What do nurses look like who are thought to be good critical thinkers?

Initially I am tempted to say that they look like they know what they are doing! This highly visual society makes many assumptions and conclusions based on

TABLE 3.2: Comparison of Critical Thinking Skills and Dispositions

Comparison of Critical Thinking Skills

APA Delphi study	*Nursing Delphi study*	*Watson-Glaser Measures*
Inference	Information seeking	Inference
Analysis	Analyzing	Recognition of assumptions
Explanation	Discriminating	Deduction
Interpretation	Predicting	Interpretation
Evaluation	Applying standards	Evaluation of arguments
Self-regulation	Logical reasoning	Transforming knowledge

Comparison of Critical Thinking Dispositions

The Ideal Critical Thinker (APA Delphi Study)	*Habits of Mind* (Nursing Delphi Study)
Truth seeking: desire for the best knowledge, even if it does not support one's own beliefs	**Intellectual integrity:** seeking the truth even if the results are contrary to one's beliefs
Open-minded: tolerant of divergent views	**Open-minded:** receptive to divergent views
Analytical: reason and evidence, alert to problems, and anticipating consequences	**Reflection:** contemplating one's assumptions for deeper understanding and self-evaluation
Systematic: valuing organization, focus, and diligence to problem approach	**Perseverance:** determination to overcome obstacles
Self-confidence: in own reasoning skills	**Confidence:** in one's reasoning
Inquisitive: eager to acquire knowledge	**Inquisitive:** thoughtful questioning, eagerness to know
Maturity: in making, suspending, and revising judgments	**Contextual perspective:** consideration of whole situation and relevancy to some happening
	Creativity: imagining alternatives
	Flexibility: capacity to adapt
	Intuition: insightful sense of knowing

looks, and it is no secret that the more attractive and well groomed individual is thought to have at least 25 more IQ points than the one who does not look as well put together. While that may not seem "fair," or even true, it is the cultural component of our society and, as critical thinkers, we need to be aware of those underlying perceptions.

On the other hand, I think it is very important to have that visual mindset, so that when you recognize the behavior in other colleagues and staff, you can call attention to it and offer the positive feedback that will continue to reinforce the desired approaches. You might learn a new approach or two, as well!

Beeken (1997) conducted a study of nurse managers and nurses to get a real life description of nurses demonstrating critical thinking behaviors. In the descriptions of the "exemplary nurse," the following traits were observed:

- Independent thinkers, thinking on their feet with sound reasoning skills
- Have the intuition of knowing
- Can do crisis intervention, taking care of problems on their own
- Can think and go beyond the current issue
- Have clear, concise communication skills, making their expectations easily understood
- Likely to listen to others, and to consider input when making decisions
- Well-groomed, self confident, and "professional"

7. If there are lists of the "exemplary critical thinking nurse," what characteristics are demonstrated by the nurse who is not the best thinker? Is the behavior just the opposite?

In the same study, Beeken noted that the most consistent comment from managers describing "struggling nurses" was that "they can't see the big picture." Other traits included hazy decision making, being afraid to make decisions, and therefore waiting for others to make the decision. They tend not to listen, may talk down to others, and be more rigid in their behaviors. Most importantly, from the perspective of the nursing shortage, these nurses are seen as being less satisfied than exemplary nurses, demonstrate lack of self-care, tend to be insecure, and are unwilling to take responsibility. The challenge becomes, how do we take the time and interest to develop these nurses into exemplary ones and not lose them to other careers? See Section 4 for several ideas!

8. Are there tests to determine if I am a critical thinker, and how well I do at the skill?

The formal assessment of critical thinking is limited to a very few professional areas, such as the humanities and education. Because defining the concept is still debatable, testing for critical thinking has been restricted and will continue to be until there is more research and empirical evidence to support what critical thinking actually is in specific contexts.

However, that is not to say that there are not tests available. Experts Goodwin Watson and Edward Glaser started the ball rolling with their *Critical Thinking Appraisal* developed and published in the mid 1980s. Originally designed as a tool for measuring undergraduate education effects on reasoning skills, the tool has become a benchmark for further assessment. The test has been refined and adapted to multiple uses, including employment screening, and is now available on the Internet (**http://www.psychcorpcenter.com**).

9. What about tests specific to nursing? I know that the National League for Nursing Accreditation Commission (NLNAC) required degree programs to evaluate critical thinking.

Yes, NLNAC has required accredited nursing programs to measure the development of critical thinking skills in students, and to provide evidence of the concept as a continual thread throughout all nursing courses. However, at the same time that this requirement was formalized, no consensus definition was identified, and schools were left on their own to define and create measurements. Very recently, NLNAC has changed that decision, and is no longer making critical thinking measurement a requirement. See more discussion about this topic in Section 2, Chapter 6, regarding NLNAC mandates.

As a result of the NLNAC mandates, there was a tremendous entrepreneurial response, and many companies formed to create testing programs. Among these are Educational Resources (**www.eriworld.com**) and InterEd, Inc. (**www.intered.com**).

10. Are there any indicators of critical thinking that I could look for in my staff and myself?

For that answer, the expert Rosalinda Alfaro-LeFevre has the following response:

"Critical Thinking Indicators (CTIs) are short descriptions of behaviors that demonstrate the knowledge, characteristics, and skills that promote critical thinking. Because we can't read minds, we have to look at how people behave—what they *do and say*—to get an idea of what or how they think." The CTIs in Table 3.3 include behaviors addressed by several key authors and organizations (see Resources) as well as behaviors gleaned from the literature and from staff and expert nurses. They have been carefully revised over an 18-month time frame, based on expert comments. They give a picture of what it takes to think critically, making the concept of critical thinking more explicit, thus providing a tool that promotes teaching and self-improvement. Because clinical evaluation is a complex, sensitive issue, work is underway to determine how the CTIs can best be used to facilitate evaluation.

It's important to remember that these behaviors are the *ideal*. There is no perfect critical thinker. Also, remember that the behaviors listed in the comprehensive list of indicators (see Table 3.3) focus on *clinical nursing* and critical thinking from a *nursing* perspective (for example, the importance of being healthy and managing stress in the indicators is included—something not seen in the literature, but really quite obvious from a nursing perspective).

11. Which personality type is the best for critical thinking?

I think this lends itself to all kinds of interesting questions. Since we do not have complete agreement on the defining empirics of critical thinking, and only a list of generic skills that would fit several cognitive processes, it would be presumptive to consider that one personality type might be better suited to critical thinking than another.

There are all kinds of personalities, and an equal number of tests that can tell you anything you want to know. Using "personality testing" as a search word on the Internet will yield multiple tests, guaranteed to determine your personality and predisposition. While many of these may be fun, they may not be well founded in terms of research or scientific implication. (Remember to challenge the data, and your assumptions!) Of all those available, the Meyers-Briggs (MBTI®) is one of the more famous, and is readily found on the official Web site at (**http://www.aptcentral.org**).

12. Thinking takes too much time and I like to just use my gut instincts. This never seems to fail, so why should I do anything different in terms of critical thinking?

Being in tune with your "gut" is an important part of critical thinking. Since I based my doctoral study on the process of intuition, I would be the first to support any activity that increases self-awareness and helps you be more in touch with what is happening in terms of predictability. You note that "this never

TABLE 3.3: Examples of Critical Thinking Indicators™ (CTIs)™

CTIs™ Demonstrating Required Knowledge

Clarifies:

- nursing versus medical responsibilities
- signs and symptoms of commonly encountered problems and complications
- related anatomy, physiology, and pathophysiology
- reasons behind interventions, medications, and diagnostic studies
- policies and procedures and reasons behind them
- nursing process and research principles
- ethical and legal principles
- spiritual and cultural concepts

CTIs™ Demonstrating Characteristics of Critical Thinkers

Self-Confident: expresses ability to think through problems and find solutions

Inquisitive: seeks reasons, explanations, and new information

Honest and Upright: speaks and seeks the truth, even if the truth sheds unwanted light

Alert to Context: looks for changes in circumstances that may warrant a need to modify thinking or approaches

Open and Fair-Minded: shows tolerance for different viewpoints; questions how own viewpoints are influencing thinking

Analytical and Insightful: identifies relationships; shows deep understanding

Logical & Intuitive: draws reasonable conclusions (if this is so, then it follows that...because...); uses intuition as a guide to search for evidence

Reflective and Self-Corrective: carefully considers meaning of data and interpersonal interactions; corrects own thinking; observes mistakes; identifies ways to prevent mistakes

Sensitive to Diversity: expresses appreciation of human differences related to values, culture, personality, or learning style preferences; adapts to preferences when feasible

CTIs™ Demonstrating Intellectual Skills

Nursing process and decision–making skills:

- assesses systematically and comprehensively
- recognizes assumptions and inconsistencies
- checks accuracy and reliability
- identifies missing information
- distinguishes relevant from irrelevant
- supports conclusions with facts (evidence)
- sets priorities/makes decisions in a timely way
- determines outcomes specific to each patient
- reassesses to monitor responses and outcomes

Note. From *Critical thinking and clinical judgment: A practical approach* (3rd ed., pp. 46–47), by R. Alfaro-LeFevre, 2003, Philadelphia: W.B. Saunders. Copyright 2003 by W.B. Saunders.

seems to fail," and most research would support that in terms of the reflection of people who agree that the times they did not listen to their gut are the times they made choices that later did not seem to be the best. That being said, I would also suggest that in this life and death business of healthcare, the stakes are a bit higher than they might be in the field of commerce, or other industries, and so other means of decision making should also be used.

There is interesting recent research regarding clinical decision making of nurses (Lauri et al., 2001), which concluded the following: "participants working in short term care, with a high level of education, adequate work experience (5–10 years) and using both practical and theoretical (intermediate) nursing knowledge, used intuitive decision making" (p. 89).

13. Many times I just know what to do next for the patient, and yet I cannot explain it. Is this critical thinking?

Similar to the question above, we are talking about intuition, or that sense of knowing based on knowledge that may not be at the conscious level. This tacit knowledge may come from experience and a sense of connection with similar circumstances, and the physiologic alert may be a sense of apprehension felt in the gut or on the back of the neck. (Just as critical thinking has controversial definitions, intuition suffers the same difficulties. I am not using intuition in this context as a psychic ability, or the ability to know something without evidence.)

As noted in the questions regarding behaviors, skills, and habits of mind, intuition is a consistent component. Benner (1999) recognized intuition in the development of the expert practitioner, and is now referring to the process as clinical forethought. "Knowing" the patient is a concept used to describe that information that comes through a relationship with another, and the relevance and connection that information has to the myriad of experiences already compiled to make up your store of knowledge.

Carper's (1978) classic fundamental ways of knowing identified four patterns of synthesizing knowledge: empirics, esthetics, personal knowledge, and moral knowledge. To be able to identify the significance of a patient's behavior and then determine what need is being expressed, is certainly the art of nursing. It is also the process of critical thinking, as we examine the subjective data, make a comparative analysis, and relate to the patient, all through the filters of personal and moral knowledge, as we come to "know" the patient. What better demonstration of the esthetics of critical thinking?

14. The workforce is aging, and the average age of practicing nurses is about 47 or so. Does age affect their thinking, and are they better at it because of their age and experience?

I tend to agree with the research and the experts, and subscribe to the use it or lose it theory, believing that if you keep active and engaged, you can reap the full benefits of a growing foundation of experience. Consider the Supreme Court judges, the oldest of whom is 82, while others are in their seventies. We have had presidents in their seventies as well, so there are plenty of examples to demonstrate that thinking capacities do not have to diminish because of aging. Gene Cohen (2000), a geriatrician and psychiatrist, does an excellent job discussing aging as an exciting opportunity. I would recommend reading his book to anyone who is dismayed by the "effects of aging." He cites numerous examples of people winning awards, publishing books, and doing their best work later in life. Consider Frank Lloyd Wright designing the Guggenheim Museum at the age of 92; Golda Meir being the Prime Minister of Israel at the age of 70; Geronimo writing his autobiography at 77; and Sir Isaac Newton publishing the third edition of his calculus masterpiece at the age of 84. It seems like a nurse at 47 is just a youngster in this esteemed company!

We would do well to remember that the brain is the only resource that is not diminishing in this day and age. Consider that all other natural resources are in some way being consumed, and it is apparent that there is good reason for the recent increase in efforts to look within and further develop the one resource that will profoundly affect all others. What an exciting time!

15. On the other hand, what do age and experience have to do with nursing, in terms of critical thinking abilities?

No doubt the work of Patricia Benner and the development of the novice to expert theory that is used as the hallmark of becoming comes to mind. Benner's work, and that of others, determined that there are behaviors that are part of each stage of advancement, and that age and experience play influential roles in the process. There appears to be a law of diminishing returns, however; one must be sure to consider both the age and the quality of experience. There are nurses who remain in one role for a number of years, and appear to be doing things the same way they did when first starting. Thus, a nurse with 20 years of experience in the same position may have learned and advanced all he/she was going to within the first year, and then simply has repeated that same year over and over again. A different nurse, electing to remain in the same position, may take the opportunity to become active outside of the confines of the role, become involved in a national professional organization, and attend many lectures or workshops to continue growth and development as an expert clinician. While the latter nurse remains in the same role of employment, has additional experience outside the role had a positive influence on the ability to think critically? I am not sure how that would be measured, and would tend to make the assumption, based on personal experience, that the latter nurse would have greater critical thinking abilities.

Regarding age, one thinks of the maturity factor and, from that standpoint, assumes that the older individual may have more wisdom, and, therefore, is more likely to be a critical thinker than the youngster just entering college. Certainly life's experiences affect the richness of our foundation, but only if we choose to pay attention and to maximize all of the learning opportunities available.

16. If we consider age and experience, what about education? Does more education make you a better critical thinker?

Schutzenhofer and Musser (1994) have done considerable work in the field of nursing autonomy, developing a tool to assess staff perceptions regarding the ability to make decisions independently in the clinical field. Numerous studies show a mixed correlation between educational levels in nursing and the sense of autonomy that is perceived. In my own assessments using the tool, I have found the same mix of responses and have not been able to make a consistent link between age, years of experience, education, and the sense of autonomy perceived.

In terms of intuitive practice, the research I have done also did not demonstrate a significant link to age and experience, other than the new graduate. There were nurses who demonstrated reluctance to act on intuitive insights, despite over 20 years of experience, just as there were those with less than 10 years of experience who stated that nothing ever got in their way in terms of caring for the patient. New graduates, those with less than two years of experience, shared reluctance to take any action, and generally scored lower on the autonomy test as well.

Lauri and colleagues' (2001) study of decision making demonstrated that analytical decision making (as opposed to the higher level of intuitive decision making) was more characteristic of the nurses working in long term care, with lower level of education, and either short (< 5 years) or long (> 10 years) experience.

17. What about those who are just starting in nursing? Are they critical thinkers because they just finished school?

A novice nurse is more likely to employ beginning analytical approaches to problem solving and not have the depth of experience and awareness to draw upon in terms of tacit knowledge, moral maturity, or contextual understanding. However, it will again depend upon the individual. There are many new grads who are in second career choices, much older than the 20–21-year-old who has progressed from high school through a college degree program. I have found that the individual returning to school later in life, perhaps after the children are grown or changing careers in the mid 30s or 40s, may still be a new grad in terms of the discipline of nursing, but may also have much more refined thinking and reasoning developed in her first career.

So, as an overlay, the individual might be very skilled in the general process of critical thinking, and still have a novice approach in the discipline of nursing. The novice and advanced beginner make clinical decisions on one issue at a time. They focus narrowly on limited, sometimes irrelevant, information. They lack the knowledge and experience to see a pattern, or a bigger picture. Therefore, they reason simplistically. And as a result, they may either come to conclusions quickly, or may continue to seek one more piece of data and be reluctant to come to a conclusion because they lack confidence and feel uncertain.

For example, a nurse at this stage of development may observe that an elderly patient seems confused this morning. She may note the patient's complaint of light-headedness and weakness. The nurse may immediately decide that the patient is presenting a transient symptom of the aging process and conclude only that she will need assistance to help the patient out of bed. Or, she may decide that she needs more information. She looks at the a.m. blood glucose. She reviews the medication profile with special attention to PRN medications. She looks for evidence of dehydration. But after collecting all of this information, she is uncertain what these findings imply and still considers that perhaps she needs to call the physician because the patient may have suffered a CVA.

A very simple example that illustrates the stage of development is when a nurse expresses alarm at a single lab finding (e.g., serum glucose = 60). And yes, that's alarming, but it may be an upward trend and expected response to treatment for insulin shock.

18. We have talked about age, education, and experience. Are there other factors that affect/influence my ability to think critically?

I use this as a leading question in discussion groups as it is one way to get people thinking about what affects them, from the environment, to the way they are feeling personally, to the type of work they are doing. Self-awareness is one of the fundamental attributes of a critical thinker, as we have noted, and it is important to take every opportunity to heighten that sense of awareness. Too often, I find that nurses deny themselves the time or occasion to consider personal impact and effectiveness. For example, when admitting a patient, it would be very helpful for the nurse to consider how that particular individual is affecting her—does this new patient make me feel intimidated (he is a personal injury attorney with appendicitis), does he make me feel sad (he is a quadriplegic with a young child, and has just been divorced), or does he make me feel frustrated (he is a COPD patient who only wants to smoke, despite continued warnings)? Too often, we are not in touch with these factors, and are taught to ignore or deny them, only to see them surface in coffee break discussions and passive aggressive behaviors.

I would suggest that you consider both personal and organizational or situational factors that are part of the practice of nursing and see what kind of list you generate. Certainly time constraints, resources, personal health, and emotional state (e.g., tired, excited, stressed) will make the list.

19. Are there things that I can do to improve my thinking?

There is the current popular opinion that is supported by research that the brain is like a muscle. As such, it will atrophy without use, and will improve with continued use. In the most recent decade of the nineties, known as "the decade of the brain," there were more studies done to validate what the philosophers have told us centuries ago about how the brain works. As baby boomers age, the significant issue of concern is the possibility of having Alzheimer's and thus, this is an area of considerable study. From these ongoing studies, we have further validated the premise that you need to "use it or lose it" and are busy creating tools and ideas that will forestall the early onset of senility or impaired cognitive functioning.

Some of the ideas that have surfaced in recent years are discussed at the Web site:

www.keepyourbrainalive.com

At this site, two behavioral psychologists suggest 83 different exercises for "neurobics" with the idea that doing simple habitual tasks differently will stimulate the brain to form new pathways, and this exercise results in better brain functioning. Ideas such as brushing your teeth with the non-dominant hand, getting in the car and starting it with your eyes closed, and wearing your watch on the other hand are simple ways of challenging the brain to get out of its rut. Have fun!

TV is also a "no-brainer" and has been found to be causing damage in terms of turning off the brain. It would no doubt depend on the program, but there is wisdom in limiting TV viewing to a select few programs. Try word games like Scrabble and anagrams instead, and try crossword puzzles as well.

20. Are there certain people who are more apt to think critically? How would I know if I am one?

I would think that those individuals who have some of the skills of critical thinkers would be more apt to approach issues and problems from a critical perspective. However, that then leads one to think in terms of stereotypes and quickly flies in the face of critical thinking. When we say someone is born to be a nurse, what picture comes to mind? Is it the feminine, soft-spoken, caring individual who has a pleasing personality? Then what about the man who is direct, communicates his intentions clearly and reasonably, and has a scientific approach to problems, always seeming to get things done in an efficient and effective manner? Who is the critical thinker, and who is the best nurse?

We could have all kinds of interesting discussions, and I recommend this for thinking out of the box and getting people to be more open to other perspectives. Consider, is an artist a critical thinker? What about the concert violinist opening at Carnegie Hall (but she is only 14!)? And how about the local florist who does the most original arrangements for special occasions? Is the President a critical thinker? What about Robert Frost or Maya Angelou? How about Oprah or Martha Stewart? Was Florence Nightingale?

RESOURCES

Alfaro-LeFevre, R. (2003). *Critical thinking and clinical judgment: A practical approach* (3rd ed.). Philadelphia: Saunders.

Beeken, J. (1997). The relationship between critical thinking and self-concept in staff nurses and the influence of these characteristics on nursing practice. *Journal of Nursing Staff Development, 13*(5), 272–278.

Benner, P. (1999). *Clinical wisdom & interventions in critical care.* Philadelphia: Saunders.

Carper, B. (1978). *Fundamental patterns of knowing in nursing.* Gaithersburg, MD: Aspen.

Cohen, G. D. (2000). *The creative age.* New York: Avon Books.

Lauri, S., Salantera, S., Chalmers, K., Ekman, S. L., Kim, H. S., Kappeli, S., & MacLeod, M. (2001). An exploratory study of clinical decision making in five countries. *Journal of Nursing Scholarship, 33*(1), 83–90.

Scheffer, B. K., & Rubenfeld, M. G. (2000). A consensus statement on critical thinking in nursing. *Journal of Nursing Education, 39*(8), 352–359.

Schutzenhofer, K. K., & Musser, D. B. (1994). Nurse characteristics and professional autonomy. *Image: Journal of Nursing Scholarship, 26*(3), 201–205.

Chapter 4: Critical Thinking Models and Their Application

> *"The significant problems we face cannot be solved at the same level of thinking we were at when we created them."*
>
> —Albert Einstein

1. Most adults are visual learners, and a model helps to clarify a process. Are there models to help with the development and defining of critical thinking?

Indeed, most of us benefit from some illustration or pictorial device that will help clarify what might be a confusing concept. The difficulty lies in the consideration that one might use the model as a roadmap and never deviate from the steps outlined. This would certainly limit the development of critical thinking and could instead create a rigid process that all adhere to without exception, and thereby miss opportunities to see things differently and consider all perspectives. I do not know of any one model that would be a perfect application at all times and would suggest that models are a good "jump start," or process to begin, and then move on to a more progressive, open-ended process of thinking. However, these are not really models of critical thinking in its totality, but represent ways of looking at problem solving and making decisions.

2. I understood that using any model is counter to the concept of creativity and critical thinking. Should a model be used at all?

There is great debate that the use of a model will limit the opportunity to think in all dimensions, and will simply create a linear track on which to go down when considering a problem. I believe that the nursing process is a good model, and an excellent place to start in terms of structuring the learning/thinking processes of the novice practitioner and student. I would also suggest that other models have their merit as well, depending on the situation. Airline pilots use a check list to order their thinking before take off and landing— two of the most stressful times in air travel when the stakes are high and the cost of error is great. These same trained pilots, no matter the degree of experience, use a checklist in times of emergencies for the same reason. In much the same way, we establish protocols for emergencies, such as the advanced cardiac life support (ACLS) logarithms. While these are prescriptive guides, they are the result of critical thinking processes, and a continued review of their application and effectiveness continues to improve their usefulness.

3. Which model is the best?

I am not sure there is any "best" model, but I would look for one that includes several dimensions and covers the questions regarding the validity of assumptions and data and assists in determining what the desired outcome is, as well as what the problem/issue/barrier might be. The two models (see Tables 4.1 and 4.2) that I have developed and used are included here as examples of what a beginning process might look like. Both have been used successfully to orient nurses in acute care, and students as well, in the development of critical thinking problem solving skills. The four-step process (see Table 4.1) includes some of the same ideas and tactics as the overall "Critical Thinking Model" and is patterned after Carl Jung's model of typology.

4. Many of the models of problem solving that I have worked with begin with an assessment in order to fully identify the data that define the issue. You include a frame of reference as well. What is this about?

I believe in the old adage, what you see depends on where you sit. As critical thinkers, we need to be fully aware of the boundaries of our individual perspectives. Without recognizing these boundaries, we cannot hope to step beyond them, to go outside of the box of our perceptual limits, and to develop a full appreciation for other perspectives.

In step one of the Critical Thinking Model (see Table 4.2), the frame of reference is clarified by shift and position. I would agree that there are very different perceptions of any situation based on the shift (day, evening, night, and even weekends only) as well as the position (e.g., staff, manager, educator, temporary worker) that an individual holds. I would also consider the environment in which one works, the organizational culture (this affects behavior and expectations), as well as the type of patients for which care is being provided. If the problem is as large as a professional focus, for example, multistate licensure, then the perspectives of home health nurses, acute care nurses, and telephone advice nurses may vary considerably and all will need to be considered.

5. Besides the obvious shift and position differences, are there other aspects to consider in the frame of reference?

I like to also include three additional aspects that are a bit more global in concept, and are sometimes overlooked, but can have a profound impact on a person's view. Consider:

- **WIIFM: What's In It For Me?:** While this may seem rather self-centered, it is a very important consideration, as it is basic human nature to look at things

TABLE 4.1: Four Steps for Problem Analysis©

Step One: Assessment—Getting the picture

Analytical: Gather specific data for an accurate, objective, and complete description of the current situation. The goal is to create a mental and verbal picture of what is happening now.

Intuitive: What does your gut say about the situation? Is there a sense of imminent danger or a "feeling" that something is about to change in either the patient or the circumstance?

Creative: What is *good* about the current problem or circumstance? List three aspects that are positive about this situation.

Reflective: How does the circumstance make you feel? What attitudes and assumptions are you using to evaluate and interpret the current condition? Is this the way you usually respond?

Step Two: Problem Definition—What's the point?

Analytical: State the problem in definitive terms, being as specific as possible, and thinking in terms of potential achievable outcomes.

Intuitive: What do you *know* about the issue, and how do you know it? Is it past experience, a reminder of a similar event, or a similarity to a problem you have faced previously?

Creative: Describe the problem as if you are explaining it on the ten o'clock news.

Reflective: How can you help others who are involved to help themselves in terms of changing the current condition to a more desired state? Ask them, "What is the most important thing that you would like to see happen?"

Step Three: Interventions and Options—Creating the plan and the part to play

Analytical: Think in terms of short term, what needs to be done now, and in the long term, what can be reviewed and clarified so that this does not repeat itself. Determine three strategies for possible solution.

Intuitive: What is your *immediate* reaction to the description of the situation?

Creative: Suspend judgment, and consider three options as if there were unlimited resources.

Reflective: What is your part in this process, and do you need anyone else to help? What will happen if you choose to do nothing? What will happen if you take action?

Step Four: Evaluation—Celebrating the success of achievement and learning

Analytical: What are the measurable effects of the actions taken? If they are positive, what actions will continue this forward progress? What has been learned from this specific event and are there future applications?

Intuitive: Consider, does this seem like the *right* thing to have done?

Creative: Identify three things that can be done to make this outcome more visible.

Reflective: Are you satisfied with your role in this process? What would you do more of next time, and what would you do differently?

TABLE 4.2: The Critical Thinking Model aka Positive Problem Solving

1. **What signs tell you that something is wrong here?**
   What is the *exact nature* of the problem, incident, or error?
   Be specific. Consider the:
   - frame of reference (e.g., your shift, position)
   - attitude (do you have a personal investment or bias?)
   - assumptions (have you verified the evidence?)
   - reasons that this problem may exist

2. **What is good about this situation?**
   Identify three aspects of the situation that are positive.

3. **What should be happening instead of what did happen?**
   These are the criteria for success.
   Be specific and measurable in defining desired outcomes so that you know when you have solved the problem.

4. **Define the problem.**
   What issue(s) are you trying to solve?

5. **To determine accountability and ownership, ask yourself:**
   - Does it affect me, patients, or team goals?
   - What will happen if I don't do something about this?
   - What could happen if I do?
   - Should I be solving this problem, or do I need someone else?

6. **What can be done about it?**
   Consider three possible solutions in terms of:
   - immediate corrections of the *short term* problem
   - *long term* remedies so the situation does not occur again
   - people/departments/systems/resources which need to be involved
   - a timeline for evaluation
   - the side effects of the proposed solution on other departments

Note: From *Clinical Delegation Skills* (p. 321), by R. Hansten and M. Washburn, 1998, Gaithersburg, MD: Aspen. Copyright 1998 by Aspen Publishers. Adapted with permission.

through our own personal filter of how this affects us. Every nurse will translate a memo from management into how this fits personally, whether it is a change in benefits, a new policy to learn and implement, or a new admit coming from ER. If the budget needs adjusting and the mileage reimbursement for travel for the home health nurse is going to be reduced by 10%, the critical thinking nurse will consider the personal impact, and perhaps look at suggesting other alternatives for economy, or changing assignments in order to reduce travel between visits. This criterion also addresses the idea of motivation. It is one thing to have the skills to think critically, but one must have the desire to do so as well—see the discussion on motivation in the chapter on resistance.

- **Past experiences:** A "been there, done that" interpretation which may be a benefit as the nurse recognizes a familiar pattern and is able to relate to past solutions that were effective. However, this can also become a form of rigidity as the nurse says, "This is the way I have always done it," and is not open to considering new options.

- **Professional stereotyping:** At times we all have prejudices that can affect our point of view by creating a prejudgment that is difficult to change. If I say the word "neurologist" on a general medical unit, there are certain to be some nurses who roll their eyes knowingly, and share stories about all neurologists being godlike, demanding, and very difficult to work with. Likewise, pharmacists and social workers may share particular distinctions, as does the more general category of physician in general. To help recognize and overcome these stereotypes, I recommend an exercise of understanding, included in the Appendix.

6. When considering frame of reference, I have often heard the term "reframing." What is reframing?

We are all prone to use our own frames of reference, our filters, our attitudes, and our prejudices when considering the symptoms of a problem. How alert we are to the existence of these influencing factors is an important first step. We are often unaware of these influences, and until time is taken to reflect on thoughts, decisions, and actions that were appropriate and effective vs. those that were ineffective, we may continue to take the same path and make some of the same mistakes we have always made. Making assumptions, and responding to cues that trigger prejudices (prejudgments), is not a way of thinking critically, but is a means of reacting to what we think is a known situation.

Reframing is really a two-step process. First, you must identify when you are using a stereotypical frame that may be influencing your interpretation of the information. For example, when you are doing an admission interview on a patient who admits to recreational drug use, how do you respond? Does this information cause you to think differently about this patient now? "He is a drug user, and will have problems with the regimen here, and we will have to be vigilant with watching our narcotics. ("They always have ways of getting drugs when they want them.") He will probably be noncompliant and not be interested in working with the plan of care." This stereotypical thought pattern of prejudgment may seriously affect how you deliver care. How would you reframe this if you knew you had a tendency to think this way about those who use illegal drugs? Perhaps you would consider that he may have an altered tolerance to medications, and will need assistance with pain management following his surgery. He may also be asking indirectly for help in determining how his recreational habit will affect his postoperative course.

7. It seems that keeping an open mind is a significant part of critical thinking and would eliminate the reframing step. Are there any strategies for keeping an open mind, and not having to reframe?

The Japanese refer to the technique as "shoshin," a clean slate, the concept of approaching something with an open mind and withholding all judgment. I believe it is a learned response, one that must be practiced in order to not succumb to the prejudices and stereotypes we have all formed throughout our experiences. Perhaps the only way to achieve this is to continually check your thinking, be reflective, and ask yourself, "What attitudes am I using that may affect the way I am looking at this issue?" Some past experiences are valid, but only when measured against the current circumstance will you know if the presumption applies to this problem as well.

8. Is reframing similar to bracketing? I have heard about that technique, but am not sure what it means.

I think that bracketing is really another means of suspending judgment by separating your inner voice, your ongoing thoughts, and paying very close attention to the issue being described at the moment. When I was working with a hospital staff to implement an outcomes-based model of care, we received report from the night shift about an 84-year-old woman with diabetes with a serious foot ulcer. The wound was being treated with wet to dry dressings, changed every shift, and the patient had been on the unit for several days. Over the weekend her behavior had changed, and she had become "noncompliant," not wanting to eat, get up, or even have the window shades open in the room. The night nurse shared that she was probably getting old, afraid of dying, and just withdrawing.

She refused to have her dressing changed, and the nurse said she was probably just going to lose the foot anyway. When I went into the room to see the patient, I took the nurse assigned to her care with me, to discuss the plan for the day, and to determine with the patient the most important things to have done that shift. I found a weepy patient in the bed and asked her what was wrong. (Meanwhile, I am thinking similar thoughts based on the night nurse's report, wondering why we are caring for this woman who is resistant to our efforts, is old, has diabetes, and is the "typical" geriatric patient—as if there is such a patient!)

It was a challenge to sit down and really listen to what this woman was saying; she had so many complaints about the staff, the hospital, her family, the food, and the list went on. I opened the window shades under protest, sat down, took her hand, and wondered to myself what she was really saying. Consciously "bracketing my thoughts," suspending the tendency to brush her off as an old complainer, I asked her what was really wrong, wondering if there was anything that had started the change and had made her so unhappy. She started to cry and told me about a very painful dressing change a couple of days prior, when the nurse had removed a dressing that had dried and stuck to the wound, causing a good deal of pain. She was told that pain was just part of the procedure, and if she had taken care of herself in the first place, it would not have happened. I offered my sympathy and noted that she must be feeling very much out of control and that could be frightening. (This is a very key part of bracketing, as I was not sharing in placing blame on the nurse, a presumptive judgment as I do not know what the nurse intended or actually did, but instead focusing on how the perception affected the patient.) The patient looked surprised, said she was frightened indeed, and most concerned about what was going to happen to her. We talked about the day, and I stressed the options she had, and how she could work with both of us to create a schedule and procedures that she was comfortable with and that the staff could follow.

At this point, you may be sighing, thinking that no one has the time for that kind of interaction anymore. Let me suggest you [bracket] your thoughts, as this conversation took less than five minutes, and made all the difference in her care. So often, we rush to judgment, task in hand, and do not allow ourselves the time to slow down enough to *listen, clarify the real issues, and make a better plan*, all part of any critical thinking model.

9. I notice in both models that you recommend looking at what is good about the situation. Why?

This is done at the recommendation of Anthony Robbins, a motivational speaker whose topics include Awaken the Giant Within and PowerTalk. On his

Web site (**www.anthonyrobbins.com**), Tony advises us to look at ways to see things in a more positive light, and to challenge the right brain to be more creative, instead of letting negativity take over. When faced with a problem, I have heard staff nurses and managers alike greet that problem with a negative, "here we go again," "it never changes around here," "nothing ever gets better, so why bother," approach. Each of these comments tells of the underlying frustration and only serves to keep the negative, downward "ain't it awful" spiral in full gear. How likely is it that you will be inspired to think creatively about solutions to the newly found problem if you persist in this kind of dialogue?

Instead, challenge staff, colleagues, and whoever is involved in the situation to consider three positive things about the existing situation. The power of three has also been researched and supported as the number it takes for the brain to recognize value and importance and to get the pathways moving in the right direction.

Consider this example: The dose of medication listed on the medication record is not a dose you are familiar with, and in fact, it seems to be rather high.

You can direct your thinking in one of two ways:

A) You already have more than you can get done in this shift, and now this! Nothing is ever done right here! Now you will have to take additional time to look it up, and find out who made the error in the first place—what a hassle!

or

B) What are three good things about this situation?

1. You recognized the problem before you gave the medication.

2. You have an opportunity to correct the error, if there is one, before others make the same mistake and the patient receives the wrong dose.

3. You may learn something about new doses for this medication.

Which process would you rather support? This strategy works well in both the professional and personal setting (particularly if you are raising teenagers, and have just found the kitchen a shambles one more time! Taking a deep breath, asking yourself what your frame of reference is, and comparing it to theirs, and then determining three good things about this messy kitchen may make it much easier to deal with the offending teen).

10. Do you have an example of how you would apply the Positive Problem Solving Model?

Absolutely! Let's consider the following issue and apply the steps of the model:

As a staff nurse, you are partnered with someone from a temporary staffing agency and have not been able to find her for the past 45 minutes. Since there is more than half of the shift left, and it has been a busy day so far, you are anxious to find her.

1. **Signs** that tell you something is wrong: Your partner has been missing for longer than you expected. This places an additional burden of patient care on you, and you may be assuming that the partner is purposely missing, either taking a long break or doing an errand you do not know about. You may be recalling past experiences with agency workers and a professional stereotype of the "casual worker" may be affecting your view of the situation. Or, you might be recalling a situation in which a worker was missing and was found in the bathroom in insulin shock.

2. **Three good things** about this situation:
   - It has only been 45 minutes.
   - You have had a partner to work with.
   - Now that you have realized the situation, you can take action.

3. **What should be happening:** Communication between the partners should be consistent so that each member knows where the other is and patient care can be delivered as planned.

4. **What is the problem:** A member of the care team is missing, and the patients may not be receiving the level of care that they require.

5. **Who is accountable:** This may involve more than you as the staff nurse. You may need other members of the team, and perhaps the charge nurse, in order to continue patient care and to locate the missing team member.

6. **Short term solutions:**
   - Speak to the charge nurse about additional help, and if he/she knows where your partner might be.
   - Ask the other members on staff if they know where the agency worker might be.
   - Wait until she returns and then ask where she has been (some staff may believe that 45 minutes is not a long time, and are willing to wait)—however, does that solve the problem?

   Long-term solutions:
   - Speak with the worker when she returns and clarify communication expectations.
   - Complete an evaluation of this individual, noting concerns regarding communication and the need to clarify expectations at the beginning of the shift.
   - Review the orientation process for agency personnel and make sure that it includes guidelines for communication regarding whereabouts.

11. I read somewhere that identifying the correct problem in the first place is more than half the battle. What does this mean, and how does it relate to critical thinking?

It has been said that the person who controls the definition of a problem controls the solution. Consider the deck hand who noted that the deck was untidy on the Titanic, and went about rearranging the chairs. They may have looked great for a time, but the boat was still sinking! I think we all have examples of times when there are tremendous resources dedicated to an issue, only to find that the situation persists after all, or the "solutions" did not result in any appreciable gain. From a larger systems and organizational perspective, examples of the effects of right sizing, downsizing, and restructuring come to mind. If the problem is financial shortfall, and the quick fix is to reduce the budget by 10%, the CFO may well have solved the problem as defined, and the budget sheets may look much better for a time, but the budget cuts may also have created many more problems that you quickly begin to realize. The budget may be the most crucial problem, but the assumptions regarding the definition of what caused the shortfall need to be challenged with some of the tough questions:

- What is our mission? And what should it be?
- Who are our prime customers? And who should they be?
- How will the community perceive our actions?
- Does everyone see the situation in the same way?
- How will our budget decisions affect everyone?

12. How does problem identification work from a clinical perspective?

Consider this example in an acute care facility: As a supervisor, you notice that some of the patients with diabetes on a medical unit are becoming hypoglycemic in the early morning hours. You note from the night shift that evening snacks are not being taken to the patients, and are still sitting in the refrigerator in the morning. What is the problem? If you define the problem as "the people who are supposed to deliver the snacks are not doing their job," then the obvious solution is to notify those people, tell them the importance of this task, and make sure that they carry it out. But is that the entire problem? Once the nursing assistants are delivering the snacks, you would expect the patients to no longer be hypoglycemic, and yet you find no visible change. There are still a disproportionate number of the patients suffering from low blood sugar in the middle of the night. Perhaps the problem needs a broader definition, and could be better stated as "there are a disproportionate number of patients with low blood sugars in the middle of the night." To reduce this number (the solution to the problem as you have just stated it) you will need more data.

In carefully reviewing the patients, their diagnoses, and the routines of the unit, you uncover some interesting details. Blood sugars are drawn by policy at 7 a.m., the night shift staff gives insulin before they leave (an old solution to a previous problem of missing the administration of a.m. insulin), and breakfast is served at 8 a.m. This is compounded by a lunch service at noon and dinner at 5 p.m., the earliest in the rotation (another "solution" from a previous dietary manager who wanted to save delivery times by starting at the top floor and progressing downward). You also find that even when the snacks are delivered, they are seldom eaten and can be found at the patients' bedsides. With this additional information, are you ready to redefine the problem? You may want to state that there is *an inadequate balance of meal deliveries, compounded by a lack of desirable snacks, which is resulting in insufficient nutritional support for patients with diabetes on this unit.* The solution now becomes more balanced meal service, with an increased variety of the nourishments that patients prefer, with the goal to be stabilization of patient blood sugar levels over a 24-hour period.

13. If defining a problem is so important, are there strategies for making sure that you do not spend time on the wrong problems?

I like the description by Mitroff (1998). He categorized five types of errors made in problem identification and strategies to correct each (see Table 4.3).

14. Is it possible to create your own model, based on organization/unit/ department needs?

Absolutely! I recommend that you get a group of interested people together, and maybe do a little research on problem solving methods in order to have some ideas about what has already been created and tried. There are so many diverse and fun approaches, particularly on the Internet. Be careful not to become overwhelmed, and consider limiting your options to three or four of the varied models. You will find some strategies for inspiring creative thinking, for eliminating thinker's block, and for finding more original approaches to the same problem. A great place to start is found on the Web site (**www.met-office. gov.uk/innovation**), which uses weather metaphors to assist with creative

TABLE 4.3: Five Types of Errors in Problem Identification

Type of Error	Description	Strategy	Clinical Example
Picking the wrong stakeholders	Using only a small group, and not considering the impact on others and their opinions	Challenge at least one assumption of the primary group, and identify at least two other groups/people who may oppose the decision	Responding to Health Insurance Portability and Accountability Act (HIPAA) regulations by eliminating the patient information board at the nurses' station—this will affect more than just the nurses on the unit—who will need to be included?
The scope of options is too limited	Looking at only one or an "either/or" solution	Consider at least two different descriptions of any problem	Two nurses who are working in the same department do not get along, and one has stated, "either she leaves, or I do"— what are other solutions to consider?
Phrasing a problem incorrectly	Using only a limited set of disciplines (one) in describing the basic nature of the problem	Consider both technical and human variables	Pharmacy and lab rely on faxes for all orders, yet lab claims there are "lost" orders and orders never received from the clinic, which results in delays of lab draws. Nursing sees this as primarily a lab problem as the system with pharmacy is similar and is working just fine. Both the implementation of the technology, and the staff involved need to be assessed in terms of the process currently in place.
Boundaries/scope of the problem are too narrow	Lack of consideration of other variables	Broaden the scope of any problem to just beyond your comfort zone	The nurse is unable to reach the physician, despite numerous repeated attempts to page him.
Failing to think systematically	Focusing on part of the problem and ignoring the connection to other parts of the whole	Beware of fragmentation and work to include all of the interactions	There is a chronic shortage of linen on the medical units, and staff is "borrowing" from other units. Including housekeeping, finance, and administration/ management in this system problem will result in a better long term solution.

Note. From *Smart thinking for crazy times: The art of solving the right problems* (p. 20), by I. Mitroff, 1998, San Francisco: Berrett-Koehler Publishers, Inc. Copyright 1998 by Berrett-Koehler Publishers, Inc. Adapted with permission.

approaches to problems. The "Blue-sky" approach is an interactive tool that takes you through these steps:

1. State the problem.
2. Describe some obvious solutions.
3. Forget about it for a moment (walking away from a problem for a few minutes is often a good strategy by itself).
4. The screen then shows you a picture of something (daisy, elephant, the world, a plane, in random order). To adapt this to a meeting environment or classroom, simply have PowerPoint images or slides to show instead of being on screen.
5. Then think of new solutions to the problem based on association with the image, and this will give you a fresh perspective.

I think for any model to be critically effective, you should be sure to cover some sort of data analysis, challenge assumptions, define the problem in measurable terms, identify the goal(s), and include steps for how to achieve the solution.

15. Should an organization adapt just one model and have everyone use it?

This is a matter of organizational preference, culture, and philosophy. Let's turn the question around for a better perspective. What do you hope to achieve by introducing one model to the organization and enforcing its use? Would it be to get everyone started in development of his or her critical thinking behaviors? How do you know that this needs to be done? In any organization, there will be varying levels and approaches to problems and decision making. If an assessment reveals inconsistent and ineffective processes at work, it would be reasonable that one model would help to develop a more consistent approach to problem solving, especially in the beginning stages of development of the concept. However, if a model were introduced exclusively and rigidly adhered to, let's say as a managerial preference, then you are working against many of the basic tenets of critical thinking. What would happen to creativity, the willingness to look at things differently and to see new ways of doing things?

Perhaps a good approach would be the introduction of the concept of critical thinking, followed by a model that is applied in staff meetings and task force meetings, and then evaluated for ease of use and effectiveness. Staff could then participate in improving the model and suggesting other approaches. The goal is simply to get people thinking and freely sharing productive ideas that lead to better ways of doing things, whether it is a new policy for visitors or a better way to reduce waiting times in the clinic.

16. Questioning seems to be a very big part of critical thinking, and I have heard that the major part of it is in asking the right questions. Is there a model or a list of such questions; that is, how do you know if it is the "right question?"

If we are talking about the idea of being open-minded, and that there is more than one way to see and do things, then there must be numerous questions, and no "wrong" question. However, there have, of course, been studies and categories developed that would assist in structuring your inquiries.

Four types of questions have been established as part of the process of teaching and thinking critically (Kyzer, 1996). To illustrate their application, consider the following clinical example and the questions:

A post-operative patient with a thoracotomy is complaining of pain that is not relieved by currently ordered medications.

1. Factual:

What medications is the patient receiving?

When was the last dose?

Has the patient received more than one medication?

2. Interpretative:

Is the pain different from previous pain?

Would the pain the patient is experiencing be expected in this course of treatment?

3. Creative:

Did the patient actually receive the medication as recorded, or did someone record it in error?

Or did someone divert the drug?

4. Evaluative:

What do I believe is the cause of the pain?

Given all of the above, what do I believe I should do at this point?

17. Are there specific questions for dealing with the "big problems"–those that relate to a disease category, an interdisciplinary problem, or a system issue?

Either of the models presented in question 3 would be great. There is also a rather simple approach for getting started, and helping to frame the issues surrounding what seems to be a "big problem." The two questions I use are basic: 1) What are the obvious problems with this situation? and 2) What are the problems that are not so obvious? The critical thinking will generally be evident in the exploration of what are the not so obvious problems.

For example, in considering the population of women with breast cancer, and the problems associated with it, ask a group of caregivers (this can be a diverse group of many disciplines) the above two questions.

The obvious problems might be listed as: diet, skin breakdown, potential for infection, impaired mobility secondary to mastectomy, and coping difficulties.

The less obvious problems might include: determining when the patient makes the transition from a patient with cancer, to a cancer survivor, and how is this facilitated?

What are the events that precede this transition, and can the stigma of cancer be minimized or eliminated?

In an interdisciplinary system problem, consider the issue of transferring patients from the ER to the inpatient units.

Obvious problems: lack of communication, errors in reporting, not enough staff/time to receive report and attend to the patient, timing of transfer during report times.

Less obvious problems: How do we measure the effect of the transfer on the patient and family and determine criteria for a successful transfer from their perspectives?

How do we establish what is important to the harmony of both the inpatient units and the ER?

18. Are there different styles of making a decision? I work with a manager who just seems to "give it his best shot," and sometimes that is a risky process.

There are numerous ways that decisions are made; most progress from intuitive to analytical in nature, with the manager being more within the intuitive range. Decisions typically fall into two categories of programmed and nonprogrammed. Programmed decisions are those made by the book, according to policy, and are based on repetitive decisions that reflect a situation that can be structured. Salary and benefits are programmed decisions, and reduce the work the manager has to do in order to manage the budget. The establishment of visiting hours creates a programmed decision which may be enforced by the unit secretary, but the nonprogrammed, and therefore creative, intuitive approach may be taken by the nurse who decides that there will be an exception to the policy for a family who just traveled across the country to see a terminally ill relative.

19. What about the use of computers to support decision making? Is there a model to follow that assures success?

Computers are an excellent tool for both supporting decision making and for helping to develop the skill. Just as clinical pathways have been used to identify treatment steps to common disease processes, similar to standards of care, computer programs are used to ensure that the information is systematically managed, trends are discovered, and a decision offered based on the variables provided through the program.

Studies are indicating that there is a benefit to the use of such computer programs. One study (Lamond & Thompson, 2000) of a computer program for assisting physicians in treating patients with abdominal pain demonstrated that there were satisfactory decreases in unnecessary laparotomies, decreases in ruptured appendices, and improved diagnostic accuracy. There is so much information and data available in this age that it has become essential to create data management tools that will aid in making better decisions. While this example relates to physicians, there is also growing evidence that the introduction of decision-making models in nursing is improving both the accuracy and identification of patient problems.

20. Is there a "short form" for critical thinking when there is not enough time to follow an in-depth model?

There is really no acceptable short form for thinking critically, although there are strategies that are used as shortcuts with varying degrees of success. One such popular approach is that of using heuristics, or "rule of thumb" decision making. For example, the manager who is writing the annual evaluation of the staff nurse may use the availability heuristic—that is, to make a decision based on the most readily available information. This is usually also the most recent information, and if it was a positive encounter in the past couple of weeks, the performance evaluation may reflect that and the staff nurse will be pleased. The staff nurse will also be pleased because the manager did not remember or address the difficulties the staff nurse had with two of the physicians and the pharmacist three months ago.

The similarity heuristic is used more than we like to admit, particularly when short of time and in a hurry. If the nurse predicts a multiprivara mother will behave as so many of the other mothers who have experienced numerous deliveries have behaved, the nurse may be surprised when the patient becomes hysterical and cannot handle labor pains.

There are usually risks associated with short forms of thinking, and the following list describes some of the more common ones, along with clinical examples:

1. **Plunging in:** Reaching conclusions before thinking it through (e.g., calling the physician about the patient's increased temperature before collecting the other vital signs or doing an assessment)

2. **Shortsighted short cuts:** Relying on "rules of thumb" or inaccurate information (e.g., giving a patient Ativan to calm him down and then starting the admission history)

3. **Overconfidence in your judgment:** Not considering other points of view because you know yours is best (e.g., the lab technician who refuses to repeat the lab test you are questioning, even though the result reported is 10 times what it should be, and is really a decimal point error)

4. **Shooting from the hip:** Doing the first thing that comes to mind, in a sense of urgency, and often just to satisfy a need to take action (e.g., calling a code before checking the patient's preference for DNR (do not resuscitate), or assessing the patient who is having a seizure)

5. **Group failure:** Group think, in which the strongest presented opinion becomes the one the group accepts, despite what may be obvious errors in judgment (e.g., the entire day shift staff, led by the charge nurse, decides that the pharmacy is not interested in working as a team, and takes a passive aggressive approach to all interactions. In reality, the pharmacy has lost two of its pharmacists, is short one tech, and has not been able to recruit replacements for the past month.)

As you can see, taking "shortcuts" in problem solving tends to create more problems and make existing situations worse. There is no substitute for critical thinking!

RESOURCES

Jackson, M. & Hansten, R. (2004). Clinical delegation skills (3rd ed.) Sudbury, MA: Jones and Bartlett Publishers.

Kyzer, S. P. (1996). Sharpening your critical thinking skills. *Orthopaedic Nursing, 15*(6), 66–76.

Lamond, D., & Thompson, C. (2000). Intuition and analysis in decision making and choice. *Journal of Nursing Scholarship, 32*(4), 411–414.

Mitroff, I. (1998). *Smart thinking for crazy times.* San Francisco: Berrett-Koehler Publishers, Inc.

Russo, J. E., & Schoemaker, P. (1989). *Decision traps.* New York: Simon and Schuster.

Section 2:
Developing the Elephant: Strategies for Facilitating Critical Thinking at All Levels

As we've discussed thus far, critical thinking is innate, can be developed, and needs a positive attitude. This section discusses strategies to promote critical thinking that are specific and practical. Pre-licensure students can benefit from use of these strategies and from well written test questions. Yet staff, new and experienced, benefit from continuously challenging their thinking, keeping their clinical decision-making skills sharp. Overcoming resistance to the thought that there are no new ideas is a challenge in both practice and academia—and can be changed if we practice critical thinking ourselves.

5. **Phases of Development**
   Donna Ignatavicius, MS, RN

6. **Learning Strategies to Promote Critical Thinking**
   Donna Ignatavicius, MS, RN

7. **Critical Thinking and Test Construction**
   Kathy Missildine, MSN, RN, CS

8. **Novice Nurse Learning Experiences**
   Jackie McVey, PhD, RN

9. **Staff Perceptions and Effects**
   Donna Ignatavicius, MS, RN

10. **Overcoming Barriers and Identifying the Resistance**
    Marilynn Jackson, PhD, MA, RN
    Bette Case, PhD, RN, BC

Chapter 5: Phases of Development

> *"Intellectual growth should commence at birth and cease only at death."*
>
> —Albert Einstein

1. Is critical thinking a new idea? Where did the concept originate?

Critical thinking actually started to appear in general education literature over 30 years ago. Advocates of critical thinking believed that learning occurs best when thinking is stimulated. When I really think about how I learn best, I do believe it is when my thinking is fostered, or even challenged. Of course, believers in this idea were way ahead of their time, and it's only been recently that critical thinking has become so popular.

2. Has the general education system (K–12) been historically receptive to critical thinking development?

The education system in the United States wasn't universally open to the thinking-learning connection. Most of the teachers I remember believed in rote memorization and lots of "drill and practice." Although we all need to memorize a certain amount of information, we also need inquiry, analysis, and inference.

When most of us went through K–12 grades, we used textbooks that required us to memorize facts and look up pieces of information to answer study questions, such as historical dates. But today, you and I can't recall many of those dates because no one helped us think about why they were important and how America might be different if these events had not occurred.

Today's textbooks, though, are very different from those we had. I've seen first grade readers with "Thinking Questions" at the end of each story. It's never too early to stimulate thinking!

3. Is the general education system now focusing more on critical thinking, especially as it relates to learning?

Fortunately, yes! Most state educational systems are helping teachers learn how to foster critical thinking in the classroom. I know that in my county several consultants have provided workshops designed specifically for teachers. In addition, throughout the country there are a lot of national conferences and regional seminars where critical thinking is being taught. Dr. Richard Paul and his colleagues from the Center on Critical Thinking in California are probably the most active presenters for K–12 teachers. For the past few years, they've also started conferences for educators in higher education, with special attention to healthcare educators. If you want more information, visit their website (**www.criticalthinking.org**).

The good news for employers is that we'll soon see a different type of employee. The K–12 students and college students who are developing critical thinking as part of their educational experiences will be better thinkers than many of us were when we came out of high school or nursing school. Of course, that depends on when you graduated.

4. What about higher education—how is it responding to critical thinking development?

There's a real need for a shift in higher education from a teaching to a learning philosophy. In the early 1990s, Terry O'Banion (1997) coined the term "learning college." He believed that faculty are too focused on what and how they teach, rather than focusing on how to help students learn.

As a result of his work and that of others, educators in higher education are also trying to become more aware of how to stimulate student thinking as they learn. Unfortunately, this is a very slow process, and a number of faculty are resistant to change from the way they have always taught. But I think the movement has started and will continue as seasoned educators retire and newer, more innovative ones replace them.

5. Is critical thinking the same as problem solving or the nursing process?

Not really. There's been some debate in the literature about this issue; some people think they're the same and others disagree. I truly believe that the nursing process is a problem-solving method that serves as a stepping-stone in critical thinking development. We could visualize in sort of a developmental way, with problem solving being the first step, nursing process being a higher level, and then critical thinking being the top step (see Figure 5.1).

Some problems have only one correct answer, such as 2 plus 2. Although you could argue that there could be two apples and two oranges, so 4 might not be the correct answer, the fact remains that if you took a math test and were asked for the answer to 2 + 2, it would be counted wrong if 4 were not the answer provided.

When we look at the nursing process as a higher level than problem solving, there are options to the problems, or diagnoses, that patients have. But we tend

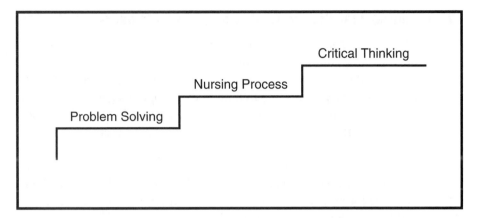

Figure 5.1: Critical Thinking Development

to plan interventions based on *each* diagnosis. For example, let's say that an older patient returns from the OR to the unit with a Demerol PCA. Several hours later, the patient is restless, acutely confused, and agitated. Some nurses would call the physician; others would assume this is normal behavior for an older adult. There is often an assumption made that the problem here is "Acute Confusion," rather than first looking at a bigger picture that might explain the behavior. What is the patient's pulse ox reading? Does the patient have a distended bladder? Is the Demerol effective for the pain? Is the Demerol causing the acute confusion? Of course, the patient should not have been on Demerol in the first place because it is contraindicated for older adults, based on recent research findings. Did the nurse question why the patient is on Demerol, and could the patient be placed on a different med?

You see, a critical thinker would consider all of those options, ask lots of questions, and look for possible answers in an attempt to see a bigger picture. That takes the care of the patient to a higher level, and ultimately ensures excellent, holistic care.

6. Why are most students who enter nursing programs not expert critical thinkers?

I addressed part of this question in the previous response about what the general education system has historically done in regard to critical thinking development. There's another factor, though, that helps to explain the quality of entering nursing students, and that is that we are not attracting as many highly qualified students into the profession.

7. Are nursing faculty required to help students develop critical thinking?

Absolutely! The National League for Nursing (NLN), which used to accredit all nursing programs, mandated that critical thinking be a part of program curricula since 1990 or so. Then the NLN Accreditation Commission (NLNAC) decided about four or five years ago to require that programs measure the students' critical thinking ability as a program outcome using reliable and valid tools. Needless to say, this requirement caused havoc because there's no one test that can fit the bill. I know of many programs that invested a great deal of money into various commercial tests and still did not get the results they hoped for. As it turns out, a decision was made in June 2002 to drop the tool requirement as an outcome for all nursing programs, although critical thinking development must still be included as part of the curriculum.

The challenge is, of course, how to really develop critical thinking in students who may come in with no critical thinking skills or little potential for their rapid development. Educators only have two to four years, depending on the program, to really help students become good thinkers, and for many, it's just not enough time. That's why it's up to employers to continue with that development through mentoring and coaching.

8. What are nursing instructors doing to help students develop critical thinking?

This is the biggest challenge for faculty, and, overall, I think they're really trying very hard to help students develop critical thinking. Some educators do a better job of it than others. In the classroom, for example, we still see some educators lecturing to students with very little interaction or stimulation of thinking. They believe that if they don't "cover" a certain amount of material, then the students won't learn it. The reality is, though, that students often don't learn it even if it's covered in class, or learning may occur elsewhere.

Some faculty further justify their actions by noting that many students do not read the textbook assignments prior to class, and come ill-prepared. Well, guess what? Students have figured out that they don't need to read because the instructor will just tell them what they need to know in class! We aren't holding students accountable for reading, or for learning, either. Somehow we have it in our minds that the instructors are accountable for student learning. And that just is not true. Students are accountable for their own learning, and educators are accountable for facilitating that learning through critical thinking activities that help students learn.

9. Are instructors generally successful in fostering critical thinking in students?

I think that they are, in general, but they only have time to help them develop beginning skills, such as learning the difference between right and wrong methods, and perfecting the correct approaches. There is no way that all students will graduate with expert critical thinking skills. That takes experience and additional learning.

10. What factors influence how pre-nursing students develop critical thinking?

The same factors apply to every person in terms of what influences critical thinking development. Personal factors are those variables you have that enhance, inhibit, or affect development of critical thinking in some way. Workplace factors can also influence the development of critical thinking for the student in a clinical experience setting. There is a terrific shortage of places available for onsite clinical experiences, and some of those chosen present additional challenges for the learning student, as the shortages of staff and the changes in healthcare delivery affect each work site differently. Table 5.1 lists some of these variables.

11. Are some people just "born to be" better critical thinkers than others?

I don't think that people are born with a predisposition to critical thinking because it can be developed in anyone. Some people just take longer than others to become expert thinkers and need other methods of development. While most of us are primarily visual learners, there are a good number who need to hear the lesson, and still others who learn better by doing. I think a variety of methods works best, and then the key is to recognize all people will go at their own pace.

I've recently become very interested in a set of skills collectively referred to as emotional intelligence, or EQ. In my opinion, and it is just my opinion with no real research to back up this hypothesis, people who have ample EQ are the best critical thinkers.

12. How does emotional intelligence (EQ) relate to critical thinking development?

Emotional intelligence is a combination of intrapersonal skills (self-insight skills) and interpersonal skills (people skills). The research shows that we are all born with a certain amount of EQ, and it is housed in the limbic system of

TABLE 5.1: Variables That Influence Critical Thinking

Personal Variables	
Thinking style:	How you think obviously influences how you critically think. Are you analytical, methodical, or intuitive in your approach?
Age:	Theoretically, the older you get, the better thinker you are, but it depends on your willingness to change and learn.
Culture:	Beliefs, morals, values, generation, and religion influence how you think.
Life experiences:	Did you have opportunities for making decisions?
Self-confidence:	A critical thinker is sometimes a risk taker.
Education/knowledge level:	It's hard to think about what you don't know!
Health:	It's more difficult to concentrate if you're uncomfortable, exhausted, or stressed out!
Workplace Variables	
Time to do the work:	Time can either enhance or inhibit critical thinking.
Organizational culture:	This includes policies and procedures that can box people in, rather than allow them flexibility to think.
Peers:	It's best to be surrounded by people who encourage critical thinking.
Management:	Is the management team role modeling for critical thinking and encouraging your thinking? Or are they more dictatorial and not open to new ideas?
Staff:	Are they supportive of the learning experience, and open to questions and new ideas?
Environment:	Are there too many distractions and disruptions? It's hard to think in an over-stimulating setting.

the brain. The significance of its location is that because it's not in the gray matter on a cognitive level, it can't just be taught in a class. It must be developed, nurtured, and reinforced over time.

When you look at the components of EQ as identified by Goleman (1998) in Table 5.2, you can see that they overlap with the characteristics of a good critical thinker.

TABLE 5.2: Components of Emotional Intelligence

Intrapersonal Skills
Self-awareness: self-confidence and realistic self-assessment ability
Self-regulation: ability to control or redirect impulses and emotions
Motivation: passion for work, energetic, and a strong drive to achieve interpersonal skills
Empathy: ability to understand others, especially across cultures
Social skill: ability to proficiently manage relationships and lead teams

Note. From *Working with emotional intelligence* (p. 318), by D. Goleman, 1998, New York: Bantam Doubleday Dell. Copyright 1998 by Bantam Doubleday Dell. Adapted with permission.

I believe that critical thinkers have to have a lot, if not all, of these skills. So, that's how I see the relationship of EQ and critical thinking.

13. Are there levels of critical thinking?

Yes, I think so, and they seem to parallel learning development. The beginning thinker is at a basic level. It's in this stage that we learn the difference between right and wrong and learn to practice things the right way. For example, if you put on gloves to start an IV, but then tear a hole in one fingertip to better palpate a vein, you're not even at the basic level. You know that the right thing to do is to use standard precautions, but chose to use a method that you prefer, not the safest method. If you were truly critically thinking, you'd be saying to yourself, "What if this patient has a blood-borne disease? What might happen to me as a result of my sloppy technique?" By the way, "what if" questions are very good critical thinking questions.

As we learn about more options and become more experienced, we start looking at other ways of doing the "right" thing, or other approaches or options. For instance, using the glove example, there are newer gloves now that are thinner and fit more snugly that allow for easier palpation of veins. There are methods other than palpation to locate a vein, including asking someone else who's better at IV starts to do the task. How you locate the vein and where you place the IV depends on what you believe is the best way for you. And that's okay, as long as the standard of care is maintained.

The expert thinker knows there are various options and approaches, and selects a Plan A (with a B and C backup) based on what he/she believes is the best way. In the glove example, the newer, tighter fitting gloves may not be available. So,

Plan B or C may be the way to get the job done. If the plan works, the critical thinker assesses that the outcome has been met.

14. What level of critical thinking is likely for most nursing graduates?

In my experience, I find that most are at the beginning, or basic, level. They've just spent several years learning and practicing standards of care and they aren't ready for lots of alternatives or options until they get more experience. Most nurses, including new graduates, agree with this assessment.

15. Why are new graduates not typically functioning at the expert level?

Very few graduates are able to function at the expert level for reasons we've talked about. I do think that some are at the second level ("it depends") because of the personal variables that we discussed earlier. For example, an LPN who goes back to school to become an RN is very likely able to function at more than a beginning level. An individual who has made nursing a second career choice may also function at a higher level, using knowledge transference, age, and life experiences to add to the ability to problem solve and reason. However, if the previous career was not healthcare-related, the new second-career nursing grad will not have discipline-specific critical thinking knowledge, and may still be functioning at a beginner level.

16. How does Benner's (1984) model of professional development correlate with the levels of critical thinking?

It is the third stage of five stages, or competent stage, in which Benner (1984) said that the nurse integrates critical thinking into daily practice. I believe that stage correlates nicely with the expert level described earlier. But, remember, Benner also stated that it takes an average of 18 months to 3 years to reach the competent level. So, we have to be patient with new graduates to allow them time to grow and develop. This is a difficult concept for some employers who think that a few weeks of orientation will make new grads the equivalent of those seasoned nurses who've been there for years. And, as you know, that's just not realistic!

RESOURCES

Alfaro-LeFevre, R. (2003). *Critical thinking in nursing: A practical approach* (3rd ed.). Philadelphia: Saunders.

Anderson, C. A. (1996). Teaching is not feeding. *Nursing Outlook, 14*(6), 257–258.

Barr, R., & Tagg, J. (1995, November/December). From teaching to learning: A new paradigm for undergraduate education. *Change,* 13–25.

Benner, P. (1984). *From novice to expert.* Menlo Park, CA: Addison-Wesley.

Goleman, D. (1998). *Working with emotional intelligence.* New York: Bantam Doubleday Dell.

Martin, C. (2002). The theory of critical thinking in nursing. *Nursing Education Perspectives, 23*(5), 243–247.

O'Banion, T. (1997). *A learning college for the 21st century.* Phoenix: Oryx Press.

Chapter 6: Learning Strategies to Promote Critical Thinking

> *"Learning and then not acting on what you learn is like plowing and then never planting."*
>
> —Unknown

1. As an educator, I sometimes get frustrated that students—whether nursing students or "seasoned" nurses—don't seem to remember things they've already been taught. Then I feel as if I've failed in some way as a teacher. Have you had this problem in your teaching experience?

Yes, I certainly have. And I think that every educator has had this same experience at some time or the other. There are several reasons why this happens. First, many of us got our positions as educators with very little or no formal preparation in how to be an effective educator. Even in schools of nursing, many faculty lack formal preparation for their role. Advanced degrees in nursing education seem to be a thing of the past in favor of nurse practitioner programs. And, just because we might have a lot of knowledge or be clinically expert doesn't mean that we can effectively teach what we know!

Another reason is that even when we learn how to teach, the preparation is based on what we've always done in education at any level. In higher education, we've used a model from England that is centuries old; that is, we've told instructors that they should stand in front of the classroom and impart information to the students (O'Banion, 1997). When you're in the teaching mode, students often don't come prepared for class. So, as an instructor, you believe that you have to cover everything, even material that should have been learned previously. This has been the standard definition of teaching. But teaching does not guarantee student learning! Learning can only occur if the student is stimulated to think critically.

2. So, what is the difference between teaching and learning?

One of my favorite articles comes from a source that's about seven or eight years old, but it's fabulous in differentiating teaching and learning. Barr and Tagg (1995) addressed this issue and have clearly defined the difference between teaching and learning. Although they discussed these concepts from an undergraduate education perspective, the same tenets apply in any educational experience. Essentially, the authors emphasized that when an educator lectures in class and gives information, he/she is using a teaching model, not a learning model. But, all of us as educators must keep in mind how we can ensure student learning as an outcome, not how we can be better teachers.

Somehow, we've come to think that if we use the latest technology, such as PowerPoint, then we're certainly good teachers. But, PowerPoint is just one educational tool, just like slides and overheads. Yes, it's neat to see pictures and words fly across the screen or fade in and out, but is that entertainment or is it helping students really learn? I'm certainly not opposed to using the latest media techniques, but these do not guarantee better student learning.

Consider Table 6.1 which further contrasts teaching and learning. Use Table 6.1 to determine what model of education you use. Are you a teacher or are you a learning facilitator? After all, we are dealing with adults, and educating adults (sometimes called *andragogy*) is very different from educating children. I've noticed that in some hospital education departments, the instructors are called "learning facilitators." That sends a very distinct message to staff.

3. I'm accountable for the students' learning, and I still don't know how to focus on learning, instead of teaching.

First, you need to realize that students are accountable for their own learning, not you! You know the old saying about taking a horse to water but you can't make it drink? Education is a lot like that. You can provide information and a lot of hand-outs, but if the student doesn't want to learn, what have you accomplished?

Students need to be engaged in the learning process. In formal education classes, like those in nursing programs, the students must come prepared for class. If they don't, it's their problem, not yours. It's hard to buy into that idea

TABLE 6.1   Educator's Role in Teaching vs. Learning

Teaching	Learning
Provides information	Ensures learning outcomes
Uses lecture as a primary mode	Creates a learning environment
Fosters competition among students	Fosters cooperative learning
Shares teacher knowledge	Builds on student knowledge

Note. From "From Teaching to Learning: A New Paradigm for Undergraduate Education," by R. Barr and J. Tagg, 1995, *Change, 27*(6), pp. 12–25. Copyright 1995 by Heldref Publications. Adapted with permission.

because we all believe that we have to "cover" more material if the students don't come prepared. But, why should you take valuable time in class to review the textbook or handout material that students were supposed to have read? Or worse, review information that they had last semester. This action penalizes those students who do come prepared and gives the message to other students that it's okay if they don't read ahead of time—you'll just tell them what the book says!

In the classroom, your job is fourfold:

- Clarify
- Summarize
- Highlight
- Update

If you successfully perform those functions, you will be focusing on learning, and not just teaching. And, you'll be making the learners think about the information. You also need to get creative in the classroom, whether it's for staff development or an academic nursing class. I have found that some nursing students and practicing nurses don't value class, so they don't come, or they come and don't pay attention to what's being said. If the learner doesn't value the educational experience, he/she won't be motivated to learn. So, the approach I often start with, even in advertising the class, is to let learners know how they will be better able to care for patients as a result of the educational experience. We all want to give the best care we possibly can and be the best nurses possible.

4. I teach in the Education Department of the hospital, and I am required by the Joint Commission on Accreditation of Healthcare Organizations (JCAHO) to cover a lot of mandatory topics like infection control, abuse, and fire and safety. I get so tired of repeating the same information over and over to the staff.

Think about what I said earlier. You don't have to start from scratch and reinvent the wheel. Can't you just summarize, clarify, highlight, and/or update this material? Can't you determine what staff already know and then build on it? How about a creative game or dyad quiz? How about a cooperative learning activity? What about self-learning modules? We must make learners think about why they need this information and how it improves care.

5. **Sometimes I help out at the school with lectures or clinical experiences. The amount of time they give me to cover the information is not enough. I find that rush through the content, and then students do poorly on the test questions. What am I doing wrong?**

> I sense that you're still thinking about providing all of the information, or "covering" the material. You just referred to the classroom experience as "lecture." Right off the bat, I think you'll need to refocus on a different paradigm for education, and it's not easy to switch overnight; you're still in the "teaching" mode.
>
> We're all faced with time constraints, and I have a few suggestions. First of all, be sure that you're helping the students learn the "need to know" information, not the "nice to know" or even "nuts to know." Because we usually know so much more than the students, especially nursing students, we tend to share everything we know and want them to learn it all, too. But, it's taken many years for most of us to acquire all of our knowledge through education and experience. We can't expect students to learn all of that just yet. Remember that the goal of generic nursing programs is to produce a generalist—not a specialist in every area.
>
> Secondly, it's especially important to have nursing students apply the information and think critically about how they can use it in practice during the classroom experience, not just in the clinical practicum. If we don't do that and just provide information in a lecture/discussion, students will have a difficult time answering application level questions on their exams.

6. **Speaking of time, I also have a hard time cramming information into our orientation program here at the hospital. They only give me six weeks to orient new grads and two weeks for experienced nurses. If the grads go to specialty areas, like OB or the OR, they do get a little more time for orientation on the unit.**

> When I've held staff development positions, I felt the same way. Today with all of the cost containment issues, it's even worse. Orientation for staff nurses in hospitals has always been two weeks, even in the 1970s and 1980s. In nursing homes and home health, it might be a few days or maybe a week. Yet, the amount of information, including JCAHO requirements and all of the technology that we're using, has mushroomed. Add that fact to the increase in patient acuity and short hospital stays and it's nearly impossible to provide an adequate orientation for experienced nurses in just two weeks. As a matter of fact, I think it's actually potentially dangerous.

I think that as educators we try to re-teach information that nurses already know but must be refined or updated. Chapter 18 provides some insight into how an orientation program should be structured to ensure maximum learning and critical thinking stimulation.

7. What are some good basic learning strategies that I can use in a classroom?

Entire books have been written on this topic. One that I particularly like for nursing education is by Fuszard (1995) who presented a number of approaches that are not only good for a classroom setting but also can be used in a clinical setting. My personal educational style in a classroom is promoting the use of cooperative learning. We know that learners often learn better from their peers than from the educator.

I love to do group work—even dyad activities. A lot of methods I use come from the general educational literature, and I encourage you to do an educational research online search (Educational Resources Information Center [ERIC]) for additional strategies. I think there are a number of clearinghouses for an ERIC search, but the one I've used is **www.searchERIC.org**.

8. I find that some nurses and students don't like group work. They want me to just tell them what they need to know and be done with it! That's especially true in schools of nursing. One student told me that she paid tuition for me to teach her, not for her to teach herself. How do you deal with that type of student?

I've decided that the main reason students want you to tell them what they need to know is that is what they're used to. In high school they were lectured to; in their "gen-ed" or pre-nursing courses they were lectured to. They read a chapter, took class notes, memorized the notes, and then "spit back" the same information on the test. There's no long-term learning of essential concepts when this method is used.

Instead, if we challenge students to think, especially in groups where they get peer support and encouragement, learning is more likely to occur. Of course, some students don't want to think, and some won't want to participate; they'd rather be spoon-fed. There was a great editorial entitled, "Teaching is Not Feeding" (Anderson, 1996). We tell students and nurses that we want them to think critically, but we spoon feed them information. It really does not make sense.

We have to make a commitment as nursing educators to not only become better learning facilitators but also to help students understand the rationale behind why and how we want them to learn. Just like us, they have to begin thinking differently about the best ways to enhance learning.

Other good resources for enhancing learning and learning strategies can be found on **www.criticalthinking.org**. On this site, Dr. Richard Paul and his colleagues have cited "mini-books," some of which are written for students and some for educators. I've reviewed a number of them, and they're packed with helpful information to help students learn.

9. So, what are some good examples of group activities that you've used?

One of my favorite exercises, and it's very simple, is "think-pair-share." In this activity, you pose a question to the entire group, ask each learner to write down his/her answer, and then have them pair up to share and compare their answers. The answers come out of their heads and are not searched for from a book or other material.

For example, one of the activities in critical thinking workshops for staff is to have them list the characteristics of an expert critical thinker by completing this sentence with as many words as possible: "A good critical thinker is…" It's really interesting to hear their reactions when they've compared and shared answers. Many of their answers are similar, but some are very different. One learner in a pair may say to another, "Oh, that's a good one!" That's the power of cooperative learning.

10. But what about time constraints? Doesn't it take more time to do these group activities when compared to just giving them the information?

Adequate time is a common concern among educators. And, no, it takes no more time. In my critical thinking example, it takes about 3 to 5 minutes for pairs to complete their individual lists and about 2 to 3 minutes to discuss what they listed. Of course, I often comment on some of their answers to emphasize key points and interject a little humor. For instance, one of the characteristics that most groups come up with is "open-minded." So, I list that on the overhead or flip chart and say that I'm sure that when a new nurse or student comes to the unit with a new idea, they embrace the idea with open arms and look forward to trying it. That usually gets a lot of laughs because they realize that is not how many nurses respond to new ideas. For the discussion period, I allow an additional 7 to 10 minutes.

Compare that total time of 10 to 15 minutes with my giving them a list that they all copy down or look at on a handout. I'd still comment on some of them, and they'd have questions. I'm sure that would take 10 to 15 minutes. So, there's no more time expended, but I think there's more learning and maybe a little more fun. I do believe that learning can be fun!

11. What are some other activities that you use?

For discussions of legal/ethical issues, like advance directives, I prefer structured controversy. Any of these strategies can be modified to meet your preference, but the way I use this activity is to have learners pair up. One person argues the "pro" side of the issue for a minute or less, and then the other person argues the "con" side for the same time period. Then, each person takes the opposing position and argues that side for less than one minute. They can't use what the other person has already said. What I think this exercise does is to help people see more than just their side of an issue. And, you have to really think critically about the issue being debated. Then I ask anyone to volunteer some good arguments for both viewpoints.

Numbered heads together can be used several ways. The quickest method is to have the class count off by fives to sevens, depending on the size of the group. Then, you pose a question to the entire group, but specify that only a certain numbered learner can answer (e.g., only answer if you're a four.)

Another way to use this activity is to pose a question and then have learners get into their respective numbered groups, like all ones in this corner, all twos here, and so forth. Each group tackles a thought-provoking question and comes up with an answer in a specified time frame. If you want, you can reward the group with the best answer with lollipops or some small treat. I find that most people appreciate those incentives.

12. What about case studies?

I've always used a lot of case studies. The advantage of a case study is that many concepts can be looked at together. Students have to think critically about how the concepts interrelate. I never have problems coming up with cases because I just think about actual situations I've encountered, either with patients or staff. If I run out of ideas for clinical situations, I can go to Medical Records and pull some charts. Or I sometimes use books that have cases in them. The Internet is another resource.

For me, the case study often replaces lecture. When you try to add a case study after a lecture, time may be an issue or make the exercise redundant.

Case studies can be used before class, during class, or after class. In some nursing courses, students are exposed only to case studies and other self-learning activities as independent study work. A few years ago, medical education adopted problem-based learning (PBL) as an alternative to lectures in medical school. Some programs give the student a choice of lecture or independent PBL.

Glendon and Ulrich (2001) wrote a book and several articles on what they call unfolding cases. This method is a type of PBL in that the students, either individually or in a group, discover the answers of a case study in multiple parts. For example, the first part of a case may be about a patient who comes into the ED with diabetic keto acidosis and cellulitis. Several questions are asked for discussion. Then, the patient may then be admitted to ICU, where another set of questions is posed. Again, the individual student or group finds the answers. The case may further proceed to the patient's transfer to a medical unit and then to home for home care.

I've found that the advantage of unfolding cases is that they help students see the continuum of care. Students are usually assigned patients at a given time in their care, but they seldom follow through with them on a long-term basis.

13. What about using case studies in the skills lab?

Another place where I really like to use case studies or clinical scenarios is in the skills lab. So often I see that students get "checked off" for selected skills, deeming them competent, but they seem clueless when they're in the clinical setting. For instance, it's very easy to practice trach suctioning on a basic mannequin. It just lies there, and doesn't cough up sputum or have difficulty breathing during the procedure. But, when the students are performing the same procedure on a live patient, they encounter unexpected behaviors or problems for which they really aren't prepared.

Two changes that can help make a smoother transition from the skills lab to the clinical setting are 1) the use of more realistic mannequins, and 2) the use of clinical case studies as part of the skills lab practice (see Table 6.2). Several companies make mannequins in the average or higher priced category that are much more like actual patients. My favorite company is Medical Plastics Laboratory, Inc. (MPL), a member of the Laerdal family of Gatesville, Texas. I visited the main headquarters where the skills lab equipment is made, and it is top-notch and reasonably priced. It's the same company that does the CPR dolls and most of the anatomical models you see in anatomy classes. MPL also has a Create-a-Lab division that works with schools and hospitals to help them determine their needs, yet stay within their budgets. And they can suggest some resources where you can apply for grants if funds are an issue. The contact phone number is 1(800) 433–5539.

TABLE 6.2   Example Case Study for Use in Skills Laboratory

You are caring for a middle-aged man who had a partial laryngectomy and radical neck dissection. He requires frequent tracheostomy suctioning and care. He is receiving morphine via a PCA pump for pain control and oxygen via a tracheostomy mask. When you explain the suctioning procedure to him, you discover that English is his second language. He uses paper and pen to communicate with you.

1. What options do you have in the hospital setting to ensure that the patient understands your health teaching and explanations?

2. How will you determine when his tracheostomy needs to be suctioned?

3. The physician ordered hyperoxygenation with a resuscitator bag during suctioning. Perform the tracheostomy suctioning and explain the rationale for each step. Will you need assistance with this procedure? Why or why not?

4. Another nurse tells you that she inserts a few milliliters of saline into a tracheostomy to loosen secretions before suctioning. Is this procedure considered best practice? Why or why not?

Note. From *A critical thinking approach to skill development and competency evaluation* (pp. 168–169), by D. Ignatavicius, 2001, Gatesville, TX: Medical Plastics, Inc. Copyright 2001 by Medical Plastics, Inc. Reprinted with permission.

I was so impressed with this company that I agreed to write case studies for use in any skills lab, not necessarily for their equipment or limited to nursing school use. In 2001, MPL published my student and instructors' manual entitled *A Critical Thinking Approach to Skill Development and Competency Evaluation.* I wrote this book for the reason I just described, and that is because students need to practice "what if" scenarios for when they perform skills. See Table 6.2 for an example.

When answering this case study, the student uses the critical thinking skills of explanation, analysis, and inference. Concepts such as cultural diversity, oxygenation, health teaching, and physical assessment are addressed, as well as determining best practices for this patient. The student needs to be aware of current research to answer question 4.

14. Can you use groups or cooperative learning in the skills lab, too?

Yes, absolutely. Students learn from each other, sometimes better than they can learn from us! There's also a technique called cooperative or collaborative testing. I believe that ACLS training is allowing this type of testing now. And, I think it's a great idea to help people learn.

When I've used this technique in nursing programs, I give the test (usually multiple-choice) to individual students first. Then, after a break, I have them return to the classroom in groups and give each group one copy of the same test that they just took individually. Members of the group must come up with one agreed upon answer for each question, and then mark the answer sheet provided. Of course, some will just sit there and not participate, and that's okay. I usually walk around the room to encourage the "quiet ones" to speak up.

The individual and group tests are scored. In my classes, I gave each student in a group two extra points if their group score was an "A." If they got a "B" as a group grade, each student was given one extra point on the individual test. There are no added points for a group score of "C" or lower. The students love the extra points and work hard to get the answers correct. But, they also learn from each other during the discussions.

Of course, there are lots of ways to do cooperative testing. You might not give any extra points, or you might give students a choice of taking an individual or group test. You have to see what works best for you, but I have found that no matter how it's done, grade inflation is really not an issue.

15. So, that means for orientation I could give the Medication Administration Test to nurses in groups or dyads? How would we know if each nurse is competent to give meds?

First of all, the test is just one measure of competence. It's really more of a safety check. You might give the knowledge part of the test as a group experience, but then another part—maybe the drug calculation section—as an individual test. When the nurse is with a preceptor, meds will be checked and the nurse will look up information that he/she does not know. With the numbers of meds that we give today, no nurse knows everything about all the meds. It's just too much information, and the drugs keep changing all the time.

16. How do I decide which strategies to use when?

Decide on one or two ideas to start, like maybe using a few think-pair-share exercises in classes, and then maybe a cooperative test or two. All tests don't need to be cooperative testing. It's up to you.

Once you've mastered these methods, try something else. The important thing is to continue to think critically about how you can help students learn, and that means you need to be creative.

One great idea for teaching fluids and electrolytes involved faculty pre-assigning each student as a major electrolyte, intracellular fluid, or extracellular fluid.

When the students came into the classroom, they had to sit in the room as they would find these substances in the body. It was a bit chaotic at first, but once they got settled, it helped them understand fluids and electrolytes better. Then, during class, volunteers from each group came forward to demonstrate the movements, such as osmosis and diffusion. Students loved this class so much that they asked that all of their classes be designed this way. And, they did much better on their unit exams than in previous years! Again, all it takes is a little creativity, a major indicator of critical thinking.

17. I have a friend who's getting a doctorate; she mentioned using something called graphic organizers. She said that Gen Xers are usually more visual learners and like to be entertained, so these were good tools to use. Can you explain?

There's an entire family of graphic organizers from which to select. Simply stated, a graphic organizer is a learning tool that presents information in graphic form (like a picture) and organizes it to help the student learn the information more easily. Decision-making trees, algorithms, Venn diagrams, mind maps— they're all examples of graphic organizers.

The one that I use more than any other is a type of mind map called concept maps. If you think about how people learn, they learn the major concepts and then the subconcepts. Then, they order them in some sequence, subordination, or relationship to fully grasp them (Novak & Gowin, 1984).

Concept maps present each concept, subconcept, and the relationships among them. On the map, major concepts are connected by lines to show subordinate concepts; and they're then interconnected as they relate to each other. They can be as simple or complicated as you make them, depending on the number of concepts you include. Figure 6.1 is a "map" of pain that shows the learner what interventions are similar when comparing acute and chronic pain. The map could illustrate pain as the major concept, or focus more narrowly on just pain assessment or interventions.

Concept maps can be prepared prior to class and shown to the group while I'm discussing the concept. Or the students could create a map, either individually or as a group. I sometimes give each group a piece of butcher paper and markers/crayons and let them get creative. This is another opportunity for cooperative learning and critical thinking.

When I've worked with nursing students, I've had them do clinical correlation maps. Instead of identifying an actual central concept, the patient's major diagnosis is the central point, and the steps of nursing process are included on the

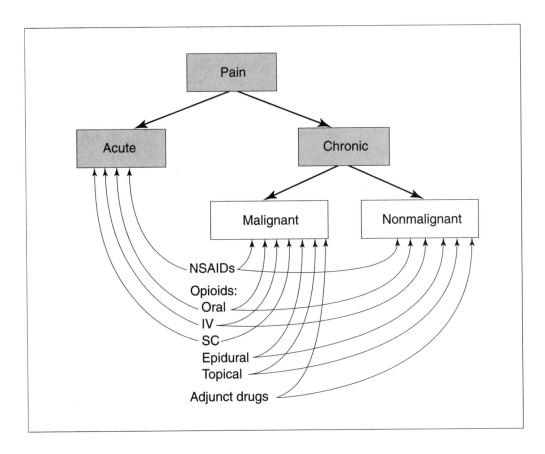

Figure 6.1: Sample Concept Map—Common Drug Therapy for Pain

map (see Figure 6.2). Connections are made between assessment data, nursing diagnoses, nursing interventions, and expected outcomes.

18. Should students construct clinical correlation maps instead of the traditional care plans they've always been required to do in their clinical experience?

Absolutely! I like the typical care plan format for the first semester when beginning students are learning the steps of the nursing process. But you have to remember that students soon learn to copy plans out of a book, and they no longer serve as learning tools. The nursing process can be a very linear process if it's not used appropriately, whereas critical thinking is more helical, presenting more of a holistic view of the patient, yet descriptive and accurate.

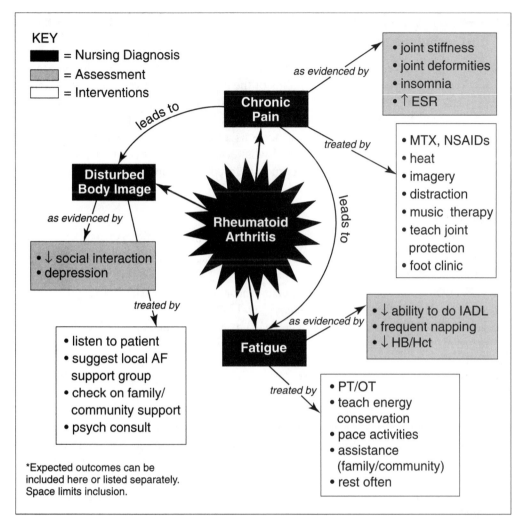

KEY
■ = Nursing Diagnosis
▨ = Assessment
☐ = Interventions

as evidenced by
- joint stiffness
- joint deformities
- insomnia
- ↑ ESR

Chronic Pain

leads to

treated by
- MTX, NSAIDs
- heat
- imagery
- distraction
- music therapy
- teach joint protection
- foot clinic

Disturbed Body Image

Rheumatoid Arthritis

leads to

as evidenced by
- ↓ social interaction
- depression

treated by
- listen to patient
- suggest local AF support group
- check on family/ community support
- psych consult

Fatigue

as evidenced by
- ↓ ability to do IADL
- frequent napping
- ↓ HB/Hct

treated by
- PT/OT
- teach energy conservation
- pace activities
- assistance (family/community)
- rest often

*Expected outcomes can be included here or listed separately. Space limits inclusion.

Figure 6.2: Sample Correlation Map—Rheumatoid Arthritis (expected outcomes can be included here or listed separately. Space limits inclusion).

19. What about grading these maps as we've always had to grade care plans?

Yes, if you want you can grade them, but I have found that it's a bit cumbersome. The 1999 article by Daley et al. described one way of grading any type of concept map. I think that the most important value of concept maps in any form is that students are learning and they're thinking critically. When they make connections between subconcepts, I know that they're thinking.

20. Can I use graphic organizers like concept maps in orientation? Or is this technique only used in nursing schools?

When you're presenting information about infection control, for example, couldn't you map out the elements of the topic to show how all the subconcepts and "rules" relate? Or couldn't you have the learners map certain concepts in groups? Sometimes I've given learners a case study and had them map the information using the nursing process as a framework. This helps them find the missing pieces of information and what else they might need to assess or determine. Visit **www.inspiration.com** to help you develop concept maps.

RESOURCES

Anderson, C. A. (1996). Teaching is not feeding. *Nursing Outlook, 14*(6), 257–258.

Barr, R., & Tagg, J. (1995, November/December). From teaching to learning: A new paradigm for undergraduate education. *Change,* 13–25.

Daley, B. (1996). Concept maps: Linking nursing theory to clinical nursing practice. *The Journal of Continuing Education in Nursing, 27*(1), 17–27.

Daley, B. J., Shaw, C. R., Balistrieri, T., Glasenapp, K., & Piacentine, L. (1999). Concept maps: A strategy to teach and evaluate critical thinking. *Journal of Nursing Education, 38*(1), 42–47.

Fuszard, B. (1995). *Innovative teaching strategies in nursing* (2nd ed.). Gaithersburg, MD: Aspen.

Glendon, K. J., & Ulrich, D. L. (2001). *Unfolding case studies: Experiencing the realities of clinical nursing practice.* Upper Saddle River, NJ: Prentice-Hall.

Ignatavicius, D. (2001). *A critical thinking approach to skill development and competency evaluation* (Student Guide and Instructor's Manual). Gatesville, TX: Medical Plastic Laboratories, Inc.

McDonald, M. E. (2002). *Systematic assessment of learning outcomes: Developing multiple-choice exams.* Sudbury, MA: Jones & Bartlett.

Mueller, A., Johnston, M., & Bligh, D. (2001). Mind-mapped care plans: A remarkable alternative to traditional nursing care plans. *Nurse Educator, 26*(2), 75–80.

Novak, J., & Gowin, D. B. (1984). *Learning how to learn.* New York: Cambridge University Press.

O'Banion, T. (1997). *A learning college for the 21st century.* Phoenix: Oryx Press.

Schuster, P. (2002). *Concept mapping.* Philadelphia: F. A. Davis.

Schuster, P. (2000). Concept mapping: Reducing clinical care plan paperwork and increasing learning. *Nurse Educator, 25*(2), 76–81.

Chapter 7: Critical Thinking and Test Construction

"Education is the most powerful weapon which you can use to change the world."

—Nelson Mandela

1. Why should exams in nursing be critical thinking exams?

We have been working to improve testing in nursing education for several years. The emphasis on critical thinking is just the next step, a refining of the process. Perhaps the need for critical thinking is best understood in the context of the growth of our profession, our coming of age, so to speak. We are a relatively young profession, and have been struggling to define our role in health care and our identity within the realm of healthcare professionals. We are currently in a stage of active growth, a state of change. A comparison can be made between the profession of nursing and the adolescent who is struggling to define his/her identity, to break free of parental control, and deal with profound physical and emotional changes. Nursing is defining its theory, practice, and place in society and is engaged in a struggle to be recognized as a profession. Nursing is also breaking away from parental control, the control of traditional medicine, and seeking to define a unique role and identity. Critical thinking is essential to support this growth, to manage the changes that are occurring at an astounding pace, and to prepare nurses to practice in the future.

The purpose of nursing education is to teach new nurses to *think like a nurse* (to borrow a phrase from Richard Paul (1998) and this cannot be accomplished with purely a knowledge level of cognition. To teach a student of nursing to think like a nurse will require not just knowledge, but the assimilation, application, analysis, and synthesis of knowledge in a variety of nursing situations. It follows, then, that the student of nursing must be continually exposed to this level of thinking, and evaluated on the ability to critically think in a variety of nursing situations.

To answer this question of "why" in a nutshell . . . we must teach nurses to think like nurses, not only for current practice, but to prepare for an exciting future.

2. It is often difficult to get individuals to defend their rationale, whether they are students, new orientees, or staff members. How can I evaluate their thinking?

A critical thinker must be able to defend a decision, and do so rationally and logically. A way to evaluate this is to ask the student to determine an action and a rationale for the action. The question may offer only two choices of actions, but give different rationale for each of the choices. Typically, a critical thinking question will vary in the soundness of the rationale. The rationale for one action, for example, will be a true statement but incorrectly applied in the given situation. For example:

> The client with newly diagnosed Type 1 diabetes mellitus has telephoned the clinic complaining of nausea and vomiting of two hours duration. She has not yet taken her usual morning insulin dose of Humulin N 15 units and Humulin R 4 units. Which advice by the nurse is appropriate, and why?
>
> A) Omit both insulins until able to take oral fluids; taking insulin in the absence of calories may result in a hypoglycemic reaction.
>
> B) Omit the Humulin N insulin, take only the Humulin R; side effects of a shorter-acting insulin are easier to manage, should they occur.
>
> C) Take both insulins, drink 1 cup regular soft drink q 1–2 hrs; glucose is manufactured by the body even in the absence of oral intake.
>
> D) Come to the clinic for an appointment; sick day situations are best handled by professional consultation.
>
> Provide correct answer and rationale. Discuss why they are incorrect.

3. Is it possible to truly test the student or orientee at the level required for critical thinking?

It is possible, but does require concentrated effort on the part of the educator. We must design test items that determine the student's ability to make sound decisions in simulated situations that mimic real-life, clinical scenarios. We must pose complex nursing problems common to a patient population, and require the students not only to take action, but also to defend their decisions logically and accurately.

4. What are characteristics of critical thinking test questions?

Critical thinking questions require the student to do more than just memorize and regurgitate knowledge. Regurgitating facts is not critical thinking. Facts are used in critical thinking, of course, but facts are not critical thinking.

To think critically, students must begin to reason, and must begin to recognize and question assumptions and inferences. Students must be exposed to the process of analyzing increasingly complex situations, and arriving at a level of reasoned judgment. Because these complex situations in nursing practice change so quickly, requiring continual reevaluation and decision making, we must prepare the student to reason in this manner. Faculty must hold students to a standard of thinking that will prepare them for the reality of the work world. To prepare them at a lesser level is, in my reasoned judgment, less than ethical.

5. How do I build critical thinking into test questions in academic as well as staff development situations?

Start by developing a few techniques, some of which are adapted from Morrison (1996). These could include 1) building "multilogical thinking" into questions, 2) requiring the student to prioritize actions or assessments, and/or 3) using distractors that require the student to employ a high degree of discrimination. Let's discuss these briefly.

Multilogical thinking, according to Morrison et al. (1996), is "thinking that requires knowledge of more than one fact to logically and systematically apply concepts to a clinical problem" (p. 28). For example, the student might be required to apply principles of growth and development, health assessment, and fluid and electrolytes when solving a problem of detecting and/or reversing dehydration in the elderly. For example:

> The elderly client is admitted with a preliminary diagnosis of urinary sepsis, with these diagnostic results: Hgb 11.2 g/dl, Hct 53%, BUN 32 mg/dl, creatinine 1.7 mg/dl, Na 145 mEq/L, K 3.2 mEq/L. Which assessment is most crucial, related to these results?
>
> A) Determine urine output.
> B) Assess tissue turgor.
> C) Assess vital signs.
> D) Obtain a pulse oximetry.

The student must know the significance of diagnostic results, the importance of fluid balance in the elderly, and the assessment parameters specific for fluid balance in order to answer the question. The nurse may have to recognize that a problem exists, draw on information from separate areas that apply to the situation, determine if sufficient information is available to make a judgment, generate possible conclusions, choose an action from a range of possibilities, or set priorities within possible actions. Not all of these, of course, are a part of every exam question, but these processes are inherent in all nursing actions, so should be tested in exam questions.

6. Where do I begin?

To build multilogical thinking into exam questions, first design a nursing situation. Create a situation in which the nurse is to make a decision, take an action, or solve a problem—then identify the thinking inherent in the situation. To find a solution, the nurse must draw upon knowledge from the areas of behavioral sciences, physiology and pathophysiology, nutrition, and socio-cultural sciences. A multilogical critical thinking question will require the student to apply knowledge from more than one of these areas, or to apply more than one fact or concept to find the solution to the situation.

Let's say that the nurse is performing a procedure and does or does not obtain the expected results. The question is based on the nursing knowledge of the purpose of the procedure, and the expected results. Then the nurse has to make a clinical judgment regarding how to proceed. For example:

> The nurse aspirates the gastric residual before administering a feeding through a PEG tube, and obtains 50 cc of green liquid. Which action should the nurse take?
>
> A) Return the aspirate to the stomach and administer the feeding.
> B) Discard the aspirate and administer the feeding through the PEG tube.
> C) Return the aspirate to the stomach and withhold the feeding.
> D) Discard the aspirate, notify the physician, and document the incident.

Answer A. This requires the nurse to know the normal volume of gastric secretions, and that these secretions are necessary for digestion. Upon the basis of this knowledge, the nurse then is able to make a decision about the next action to be taken (i.e., return the aspirate and continue with the procedure). Another example:

> The client was admitted with pericarditis two days ago. Today, the nurse has difficulty auscultating his apical heart rate; the heart sounds are muffled, and distant. Which assessment should the nurse perform first?
>
> A) Assess for presence of edema, question patient about chest pain.
> B) Take the blood pressure, assess for neck vein distention.
> C) Assess respiratory rate and bilateral breath sounds.
> D) Check for mediastinal shift and tracheal deviation.

Answer B. This time, the nurse must know that a complication of pericarditis is cardiac effusion and tamponade. The nurse must also know that accumulation of fluid in the pericardial sac will result in inability to auscultate normal heart sounds. The next step is to confirm the suspicion of cardiac tamponade by assessing for other important symptoms.

Notice that the example above regarding pericarditis also incorporates setting priorities when the questioner asks, "Which assessment should the nurse perform first?" This step is also a part of critical thinking questions. All of the assessments may be appropriate in a general assessment of the situation, except perhaps for (D), but the nurse must focus the assessment in a critical situation such as this, gathering significant data in order to take quick action.

7. Does the new grad approach multilogical tests any differently?

The novice/advanced beginner nurse tends to skip steps, moving directly to action before adequately gathering all the data. A question directed toward this tendency encourages and evaluates the ability to critically think. See the example below.

> The nurse performs assessment of the client with a chest tube that is connected to 20 cm of suction, and finds that she is short of breath and having chest pain of 5 on a 0-10 scale. There is bubbling in the water seal chamber, which was not present on the last assessment. Which action by the nurse is appropriate first?
>
> A) Administer pain medication.
> B) Palpate the chest wall for crepitus.
> C) Assess the chest wall insertion site.
> D) Document the findings.

Answer C. The nurse must first know the normal assessment findings of a closed water-seal drainage system, the signs of an air leak, and the significance of the leak to answer the question. Although relief of pain is important, the displacement and possible inadvertent removal of a chest tube would be the immediate priority. Using "document the findings" is an easy way to state that the assessment is normal and elect to take no action.

Note that each of these examples incorporates more than one technique of assessing critical thinking. The student must have several facts as a basis for decision making, must prioritize actions, and must discriminate between similar distractors. In the last question, if the distractors had referred to other body systems (e.g., percuss the abdomen or assess level of consciousness), the high level of discrimination would be lost.

8. Are there other techniques for building critical thinking that I might find helpful?

Yes, a couple of other techniques might be useful. These are 1) to require students to defend their answers, 2) to incorporate possible assumptions or prejudices, 3) to consider alternative points of view or the ability to suspend judgment, 4) the ability to synthesize data into a logical and usable manner, and 5) to take an unclear and complex issue and reformulate it to make it more amenable to solution. The question remains whether all of these can be objectively assessed in a multiple-choice format, but at least the first two techniques can be readily illustrated.

9. What are some techniques of question construction that will assess even the test-wise individual's ability to think critically?

If the exam writer is not wise to these techniques, an astute student may be able to answer the questions without having knowledge of the material. The most effective way that I have found to improve my own ability to write test items was to teach a class on test-taking strategies to students. This course was designed to assist students to be better test-takers; in actuality, it improved my test-writing skills immeasurably. The course included information about critical thinking skills, a "test-taking mind-set," components of a question, discussion of the types of multiple choice questions, and specific test-taking techniques. It was an invaluable experience, and I recommend this activity to anyone who wishes to identify mistakes in writing test items.

A few examples of "give-aways" in a test item:

A) Writing a right answer that is longer than the distractors

B) Using absolutes, such as always, never, only

C) Writing options that are not patient focused

D) Providing options that are opposites

E) Providing one global answer along with distractors that are restrictive

F) Providing options that are not within the practice of nursing

G) Using distractors that are not in congruence with the stem

H) Using identical wording in the distractor to that in the stem

10. Students say questions are too long. How do I sort out what is important, and still give them enough information?

Provide only the information necessary to answer the question. Avoid the use of names, ages (unless specific to the situation), and any patient information not pertinent to the problem at hand. After writing a question, review it to see if any words can be omitted, or thoughts expressed more concisely and succinctly. It is amazing how easily and briefly a question can be stated, and the student has a much easier job of determining what question is being asked. Consider the following wordy question:

> A 30-year-old male was involved in a motorcycle crash. Following initial assessment for injuries and immobilization of his neck at the scene, he was transported to the hospital by ambulance. Head and spine x-rays indicated a cervical neck fracture at the C5 level, and he was admitted to the trauma intensive care unit. Cervical traction with Crutchfield tongs was established. The nurse assesses him for symptoms of spinal shock. Which finding indicates the presence of spinal shock?
>
> A) Loss of motor control below the level of the injury with sensations of touch and position intact
> B) Loss of voluntary motor control but presence of reflex activity below the level of the injury
> C) Flaccid paralysis and lack of sensation below the level of the injury
> D) Involuntary, spastic movements of the upper and lower extremities

Let's analyze this question for two aspects of item construction.

- The stem is lengthy and contains considerable information that is not necessary to formulate an answer. If the objective is to identify the manifestations of spinal shock, only a simple query "Which symptoms indicate the presence of spinal shock following an injury at C5?" would be needed.
- The question is at the comprehension cognitive level, and could easily be revised to formulate an application level question. To create a higher-level question, create a set of symptoms, and then ask for indicated nursing actions. For example:

> The client, immediately following a C–5 fracture, has flaccid paralysis and lack of sensation below the level of injury. Which nursing assessment is of highest priority?
>
> A) Check DTRs, including biceps, triceps, patellar, and ankle.
> B) Determine depth and rate of respiration.
> C) Assess the abdomen for distention and bowel sounds.
> D) Determine the client's usual methods of coping with stress.

11. Would editing or rephrasing the question be helpful? Some students will state that I did not give them enough information!

Sometimes, even simple editing can result in a better question. For example, consider the following:

Original: What is the underlying rationale for...

Rephrase: What is the rationale for...

Original: An active 80-year-old has sustained a hip fracture and has had a hip replacement. The client is currently using a walker. The goal that would be most important in providing for the client's safety needs is...

Rephrase: Following a hip replacement, the client is ambulating with a walker. Which goal is most important to achieve safety needs?

12. Are there problems I should avoid when using completion style questions?

A common error consists of providing options that are not grammatically in sync with the stem. This tendency is best reduced by avoiding completion-type questions. This is an example of a stem for a completion type question, and a revision to a more acceptable format.

Original: The patient is complaining of a headache and dizziness. When assisting the patient up to the bathroom, the nurse should...

Revised: Which approach should the nurse take when assisting the patient with a headache and dizziness to the bathroom?

13. Are there other pitfalls to avoid?

Consider the following:

- Using humor in an exam. Students are not usually appreciative of this, considering the stressful situation created by testing. Humor is not useful to relieve stress in a testing situation.
- Using negatives, such as "Which is *not* indicated?" This type of question often confuses the reader and results in a wrong answer because of the manner in which the question was worded, rather than lack of knowledge of the material.
- Asking for a response that is of a low cognitive level. Formulate questions that ask the student to perform a specific action based on a principle, rather than just to know a broad principle. For example, the following is a comprehension level question:

The client with hypertension will most likely be ordered which diet?

A) Low carbohydrate

B) Low residue

C) Low sodium

D) Low protein

To change the cognitive level to application, ask the student to make a decision in a clinical situation using the applicable principles. For instance, rather than ask for the usual dietary order, supply that information, and ask the student to discriminate between food items allowed. The following is an application level question, questioning only select aspects of the nursing process:

The client with hypertension on a low sodium diet has these items on his lunch tray. Which should be removed?

A) Baked apple

B) Cheddar cheese

C) Diet cola

D) Raw carrots

I believe each faculty member has to examine his/her own habits of item writing in this area. I personally have difficulty in writing items in the evaluation stage of the nursing process, and have to check exams after writing them to determine that I have included all steps of the nursing process. An example of students' least favorite question testing the evaluation phase follows.

Which information will best evaluate the effectiveness of furosemide (Lasix)?

A) Intake/output

B) Serum K+ levels

C) Skin turgor

D) Daily weights

The students usually answer A) intake and output to this question, when the correct answer is D) daily weights. One student wrote a two-page e-mail in protest, citing all the pages in the textbook that indicate the need for I & O for the client on diuretics. A long discussion ensued, in which we explored the role of insensible loss, the inaccuracy of I & O, and the difficulty of the client's monitoring I & O in the community setting. Finally, the students seemed to have learned from this discussion and agreed that daily weights was a better answer.

14. How can I assess a student's ability to analyze and determine pertinent facts, if the stem should exclude all unnecessary data?

This is a concern of mine also. An area of particular difficulty for students in the clinical area is sifting through the voluminous data compiled for one seriously ill patient. They have to be able to gather, cluster, analyze data, and come to a conclusion in a reasonably short time. Determining the relevance of the data is a crucial step.

This degree of skill may be best evaluated with a method other than the multiple-choice item. Methods that may be more effective are case study analysis or nursing care plans. Both of these exercises require the student to analyze large amounts of complex data. I especially like to use the case study method in group settings, such as student conferences, as the students are likely to share ideas and learn from one another. It is important for the faculty member in these situations to become a facilitator rather than the teacher (i.e., the "guide on the side" rather than the "sage on the stage" approach). This allows the learners to explore options, make mistakes, and learn from their peers. This is a hard role to develop, as we often teach in the "telling" mode.

Another method, used often in conjunction with the group analysis of a case study, is development of decision trees. These assist the student to develop logical thinking, and to avoid the linear tendency of nursing process. The student uses an "if, then" approach to explore several potential alternatives.

There are some simple ways to determine if the student is able to use the appropriate data in a multiple choice exam item, at least to a limited degree. For example:

> The patient is experiencing chest pain following a thoracotomy two days ago, scored at 5 on a 0–10 scale. The nurse observes that the water level in the suction control chamber is 10 cm. The ordered suction level is 15 cm. Which action should the nurse take first?
>
> A) Administer pain medication as ordered.
> B) Disconnect the suction tubing temporarily.
> C) Fill the suction container to the correct level.
> D) Clamp the suction container tubing, and refill.

Or, give the assessment data, and ask the student to take action based on the data. An example:

> The patient is admitted with a preliminary diagnosis of urinary sepsis. Nursing assessment determined that the 24-hour urine output was 640 cc. The patient had poor tissue turgor, hypoactive bowel sounds, and 1+ edema of the

feet. An IV of D5 NS at 150 cc/hr was ordered, with antibiotics IVPB q 12 hours, and a chest x-ray was ordered. Which action should the nurse take?

A) Delay starting the IV until obtaining a report of the chest x-ray.

B) Start the IV immediately, place on an IV pump at 150 cc/hr.

C) Insert a foley catheter and place on hourly urine outputs.

D) Give the antibiotic, then heplock the IV during transport.

15. What does the instructor do, if the students just don't learn?

This sounds like the lament of many teachers, especially new teachers. However, telling is not teaching, and teaching is not necessarily learning. Although *teaching* critical thinking is beyond the scope of this discussion, a couple of comments are in order.

For learning to take place, the student must make the material his/her own. He/she must examine the material, break it down and reconstruct it so that he/she is able to derive new meanings from it, and then apply this new information in the clinical setting. The faculty's role is to facilitate this process. This can be accomplished through a variety of methods, including questioning, identifying relationships, concept mapping, constructing decision trees, case studies, group discussions and projects, simulations, and clinical experiences. In other words, the student must be actively engaged in learning and must construct his/her own understanding of the material.

This is not to say that all the responsibility for learning lies with the teacher, however. Recently, when teaching the nursing care of patients with peripheral vascular diseases in an adult health course, I cautioned the learners to review the method of measuring the patient for antiembolism hose. This was an adult health course; they would have to consult their competencies textbook for this information. When they were unable to answer the question correctly on the exam, they did not receive credit for the question. The learners did not assume responsibility for their own learning in this case.

16. If I discuss a particular nursing action in class, then test it on the exam, is it critical thinking?

It depends. Certainly, if the specific situation and choice of answers is presented in the classroom and the answer is discussed, then repeating this on an examination is not critical thinking, it is simply rote. Likewise, if the particular information is in the textbook and then asked in the same way on the examination, it is not a critical thinking question.

To avoid this predicament, pose a principle or dilemma in the classroom, facilitate student responses to apply the principle or solve the problematic situation, then present a similar (but not identical) situation on the exam. An example follows.

In the classroom, this case study situation is presented:

The client was admitted with complaints of increasing dyspnea and fatigue. A tentative diagnosis of heart failure is made. Vital signs are: blood pressure 150/72, P. 128, irregular, and R. 26. Ask the students to supply answers to the following questions. What additional nursing assessment is indicated? What laboratory data would the nurse check? What would be the anticipated approach to treatment? What would be the nurse's role in implementing, monitoring, and evaluating the effectiveness of the treatment?

On the exam:

A client with heart failure visits the clinic for a routine follow-up exam. Which question by the nurse will best determine the presence of exacerbation of the disease?

A) Are you staying on your low salt diet?

B) How would you describe your energy level?

C) Have you had any chest pain recently?

D) Are you getting up at night to urinate?

17. Is it possible to use the stages of the nursing process to compose exam items?

Absolutely! Nursing process *is* what nurses do. The emphasis on critical thinking in no way negates the importance of the use of the nursing process. Nursing process must incorporate the principles of critical thinking to be effective. Each step of the nursing process—assessment, planning, implementation, and evaluation—provides a wide range of possibilities for exam items. Inherent in each step are many mini steps, especially with the incorporation of critical thinking.

The most essential framework to use when writing exam questions for nursing students is the NCLEX test plan, as this is the blueprint for the exam to determine beginning competency in the profession. The broad categories of the NCLEX test plan are safe and effective care environment, health promotion and maintenance, psychosocial integrity, and physiological integrity.

18. How can the assessment phase of the nursing process be used to develop test items?

To answer this question, first break the assessment phase into its components. Because the nursing diagnosis is a part of this phase, I have renamed it the *assessment and diagnostic phase.*

Assessment and Diagnostic Phase

Gathering data

- What data are relevant to the particular situation?
- How are data best gathered?
  - What interviewing techniques would be most effective?
  - What assessment techniques are appropriate and accurate?
  - What data should be gathered from the medical record? From the client's family? From other healthcare workers?

Analyzing data

- Which data are normal; which are abnormal?
- What data should be clustered?
- What patterns are emerging?
- What is the meaning of these data?
- What additional data are needed?
- What inferences may be made?

19. How can the planning phase of the nursing process be used to write exam items?

To write critical thinking exam items to test the planning phase, determine first the broad categories of planning, and then break each category into appropriate subcategories. The broad categories are 1) setting priorities and identifying goals, and 2) planning interventions.

1. Setting priorities and identifying goals
   - What are the priorities of the nursing problems?
   - Which goals are appropriate for the identified nursing diagnosis?
   - Is the client involved in setting goals, and how best to involve the client?

- What would constitute a reasonable, measurable, and individualized expected outcome for this situation?
- How will we know when the goal is achieved?
- What referrals are needed, and to which discipline?
- How can computer plans of care, critical pathways, and other standardized documents be used and individualized to be applicable to the particular situation?

2. Planning interventions
   - In which areas is the client capable of meeting his/her own needs, and in which areas will he/she need nursing intervention?
   - What nursing interventions are indicated?
   - What physician-initiated interventions are likely?
   - Which collaborative interventions are indicated?
   - What Standards of Practice, legal parameters, and ethical considerations are applicable to the situation?
   - What might be the outcomes of various interventions?
   - What reassessment is needed throughout the intervention phase?
   - What equipment or resources might be needed during intervention measures?
   - What other healthcare workers might also be involved in this intervention?
   - What potential threats to safety might result from the intervention?
   - What adverse reactions or complications might result from the situation or from nursing actions? What actions should the nurse take to avoid these reactions or complications?

To write an exam item, take any of the above questions and apply it to a clinical situation. The following planning intervention example is an item written using subcategory #2 above.

The elderly client is delirious, and the nurse plans to use validation therapy. Which approach should the nurse plan to use with the client in application of this therapy?

A) Provide frequent reminders of date, time, and place.
B) Ask family members to bring a clock and calendar.
C) Assist the patient to recall events from the past.
D) Listen respectfully to what the patient expresses.

The client is prescribed corticosteroids in the treatment of inflammatory bowel disease. Which nursing plan will best prevent the development of side effects?

A) Schedule the medication to be given at bedtime.

B) Instruct the staff to check all stools for occult blood.

C) Schedule the medication to be administered with food.

D) Take vital signs, especially BP, before administering.

20. How can the implementation phase of nursing process be used in writing exam items?

The implementation phase lends itself easily to critical thinking exam questions. Consider first the numerous subcategories of implementation below.

• What nursing actions would achieve the goals?

• What nursing care can be delegated to others? What teaching needs does the client have? What techniques would be most effective?

• How can the nurse best provide a safe, effective care environment?

• How can the nurse use interpersonal skills to achieve the patient care goals?

• What technical skills should the nurse use, how are these procedures performed, how should they be modified for this patient?

• How will the nurse know when to modify the plan of care?

• What action can the nurse take, if adverse reactions to care occur?

• How can the client be best prepared for diagnostic or interventional procedures?

This is an example of a test item in the implementation phase.

Which instruction by the nurse will best prepare the client for a cardiac catheterization?

A) "There will be no pain, only a sense of pressure as the procedure is performed."

B) "You will be required to lie very still for several hours on the x-ray table."

C) "You may experience a sensation of flushing when the dye is administered."

D) "A general anesthetic will be administered, so you will feel nothing."

21. How can critical thinking test questions be constructed that reflect the evaluation phase of the nursing process?

Again, first consider all aspects of the evaluation phase, and then write questions reflecting critical thinking in each aspect. Aspects of this phase of the nursing process include:

- What client data should be gathered to determine if client goals have been achieved?
- What are the characteristics of improved client outcomes?
- What knowledge of disease process and human functioning is needed, to determine the effectiveness of nursing interventions (i.e., what are normal and what are abnormal data?)?
- Which source of data is essential to determine the effectiveness of interventions?
- What are indications that the plan of care should be modified?
- How should the plan of care be revised or modified?
- How will the nurse know when teaching is effective?
- How will the nurse know when medications are effective?
- When should a particular nursing problem be considered resolved?
- What problems might recur in the future?
- How should continuity of care for this client occur?

Examples of questions reflecting the evaluation phase of nursing process:

The client is receiving Lidocaine following a coronary artery bypass graft. To best determine the effectiveness of this medication, which data should the nurse evaluate?

A) Level of pain on a 0–10 scale
B) Level of consciousness
C) Presence of atrial dysrhythmias
D) Presence of ventricular ectopy

Which statement made by a client with an intermittent patient-controlled analgesia (PCA) pump indicates that she understands the use of the pump?

A) I can get pain medication every 10 minutes by pushing the button.
B) I can get pain medication every time I push the button.
C) I will get pain medication automatically, when I start to hurt.
D) I will not have pain, as the medicine is delivered continuously.

22. In addition to the nursing process, what other framework will assist in formulating exam questions?

Certainly, nursing exams in courses preparing the student for the NCLEX-RN exam should be written in consideration of the test plan for that exam. This blueprint is available at the National Council of State Boards of Nursing Web site (**http://www.ncsbn.org/**). The test plan is based upon the client needs for 1) a safe, effective care environment, 2) health promotion and maintenance, 3) psychosocial integrity, and 4) physiological integrity. The concepts of nursing process, caring, communication and documentation, cultural awareness, self-care, and teaching/learning are integrated throughout the exam.

23. How can I use the NCLEX test plan category, a "safe, effective care environment," to write exam questions?

The safe, effective care environment section tests the ability of the nurse to provide a setting in which the client, family or significant others, and other health-care workers are safe. This includes protection from environmental hazards and the effective management of care. This category is further divided into 1) management of care and 2) safety and infection control. Specific content areas are delineated at the Web site cited above; these would be helpful in writing exam items. An example of a test item in this category follows:

The home health nurse, visiting the home of a client with Parkinson's disease, makes these observations. Which would require immediate investigation?

A) Large pet bird in a cage

B) Throw rugs on the floor

C) Drinking water supplied by well

D) Unsecured garden chemicals

24. How can the category of the NCLEX test, plan health promotion and maintenance, be integrated into a critical thinking exam?

Health promotion and maintenance includes growth and development, and the prevention/early detection of disease. The student should know and be able to apply nursing interventions to the stages of growth and development of all age groups. The nurse should be able to recognize and prevent health problems in each age group, and assist the client to adopt health practices that sustain and maintain health. A sample question follows:

The nurse is applying for a small grant to fund a program for the prevention of the development of Type II diabetes mellitus. Which age group would benefit most from being the target of the grant?

A) school-age children

B) adolescents

C) young adults

D) older adults

25. How can the NCLEX test plan category of psychosocial integrity be incorporated into critical thinking test items?

The category of psychosocial integrity deals with the application of the nursing process to client needs of emotional wellness and social integrity of the client. The category consists of the subcategory of *coping and adaptation* activities of the nurse related to recognizing and assisting the client to manage stressful and emotional events, and the emotional and social implications of illness or injury. The category of psychosocial integrity also includes nursing in mental illnesses. An example follows.

The older adult client states "Since I've retired, I have a lot of time on my hands, but nothing to do. I guess I'm not needed much anymore." How should the nurse respond?

A) Is there any financial reason that you should continue to work?

B) You should stay home and relax. You've paid your debt to society.

C) You should get a part-time job. That would keep you busy.

D) Sounds like you like to keep busy. What do you like to do?

26. The NCLEX test plan category of "physiological integrity" seems quite familiar to me. Is that just the usual illness categories?

Yes and no. It certainly includes acute and chronic illnesses, but also includes the subcategories of basic care and comfort, pharmacological and parenteral therapies, reduction of risk potential, and physiological adaptation. Physiological integrity comprises the largest single category on the NCLEX exam, between 36–60% of the total exam. The subcategories of reduction of risk potential and physiological adaptation are the highest single categories of questions asked on the exam, with 12–18% each.

Consider this example:

> A woman in labor is to receive a spinal anesthetic for cesarean birth. She expresses concern about having a spinal headache as a result. Which response by the nurse is most appropriate?
>
> A) Keeping your bed flat will help prevent a headache.
> B) We will do our very best to keep you comfortable.
> C) Spinal headaches do not occur with our current methods.
> D) Don't worry about headaches; just think about the baby.

27. Why do I need to write rationale for exam questions? Isn't rationale provided in the textbook?

Writing rationale is an important exercise that benefits both the person writing the item, and the student in exam review. It's true that the rationale should be in the textbook, and the text page numbers may be included at the end of the rationale statements. However, when writing a critical thinking question, the rationale for the answer will not often be contained in one text reference. It will take several page numbers and possibly a combination of course textbook references to support the answer. Additionally, explanations for incorrect responses should also be given, to assist the student to "check" his/her reasoning.

A consistent format for written rationale is also helpful. For example, cite the rationale for the correct answer first, then reasons why the incorrect answers are wrong. Most of the time, it is not difficult to write a rationale for the right answer. It is more difficult to explain why the distractors are not correct, however. Avoid the tendency to write rationale as a "just because it isn't so" or as a restatement of the answer selection.

28. How can I make exam review a positive learning experience for the student? When students review the exam, they just seem to focus on arguing for points. How can I turn this around?

Exam review in this context means to provide time for the student to go back over the exam after receiving a grade, to learn from mistakes. Student exam review occurs *after* faculty has examined the statistical analysis of the exam, and made needed adjustments in grades. No adjustments are made as a result of student exam review. If this policy is adopted and made clear to students and faculty, then exam review as a learning experience becomes more achievable, as the student's grade will not be altered, regardless of the emotional intensity of a protest. The focus can now be on understanding the reasoning supporting the answers. It is best if an entire nursing program agrees to the purpose and ground rules of exam review; consistency is important to enable students to focus on learning as a result of this activity.

Exam review is ideally done in a one-on-one session with the faculty, or, if that is not possible, review with small groups of students. Avoid large groups in exam review, a situation that can easily escalate into an arguing-for-points session. A one-on-one review with faculty is ideal, although not always achievable, as this is a good opportunity for the faculty to assess the student's thinking. Students will often protest that they know the material, that their grade doesn't really reflect what they know, or that they "over-studied." But when asked why they answered a question as they did (incorrectly), they are unable to state underlying principles or pathophysiology accurately. This is invaluable information for the faculty, as it reveals gaps in knowledge. Additionally, in a one-on-one review, the faculty can assess the ability of the student to take a critical thinking type of exam, and other hindrances to learning.

29. Is it possible that the student is able to answer critical thinking type of test questions accurately, but is unable to apply critical thinking in clinical practice?

Ideally, critical thinking exams will accurately measure the ability to think critically in all nursing situations. This would provide construct validity, assuring that a critical thinking exam actually measures critical thinking (Oermann & Gaberson, 1998). To achieve this, the faculty might compare the student's scores on critical thinking exams to clinical performance ratings reflecting critical thinking. As Oermann and Gaberson suggested, however, this would require collection of data over a period of time.

An additional comment is appropriate here. Although this discussion focuses exclusively on methods to include critical thinking in testing, the establishment of reliability and validity of test items is also essential. Reliability has to do with consistency (i.e., can the results of the test be consistently reproduced). Often, testing software programs assist faculty in determining the reliability of test scores. Morrison and colleagues (1996) maintained that validity is established by the development of a test blueprint, stating that "validity refers to the extent to which a test measures what it purports to measure and is obtained through a rational or logical analysis of a test" (p. 64). The blueprint establishes the what of a test, and the importance of each category, by weighting of content. Refer to the in-depth discussions of validity and reliability in Morrison, Smith, and Britt (1996) and in McDonald (2002).

30. You mention case studies as a method of testing critical thinking. Do you have an example?

Consider the following situation, adapted from a case study written by Diane Recker in *Critical Thinking and Nursing Diagnosis*, edited by Margaret Lunney (2001). Following the situation is an example of a test item in the analysis-of-data step, requiring the student to determine which additional data are needed before making a decision. Note: This is a relatively high difficulty question.

The 74-year-old client is admitted to PACU following an abdominal procedure under general anesthesia. He moans with pain and the nurse administers an opioid analgesic. One hour later, the client's vital signs are BP 104/62, P 54, R 11. He is receiving O_2 at 32% venti mask. ABG results are pH 7.28, PCO_2 55, PO_2 100, HCO_3 26. Which additional data would best enable the nurse to determine the cause for these findings?

A) Urine output

B) Capillary refill

C) Pulse oximetry

D) Skin color

Making a nursing diagnosis:

- What are possible diagnoses for the situation?
- What are the definitions for the potential diagnoses?
- Do the defining characteristics of the diagnosis fit the current situation?
- Do the related factors apply to the current situation?
- What is the most accurate diagnosis, and what is the defense for this decision?
- What data support the nursing diagnosis?

Admittedly, the role of nursing diagnosis in the profession is considered controversial. One argument against its use is that the terminology is cumbersome. However, for the student nurse, it is a concept that can provide the needed structure for learning a commonality of language that is invaluable. It also provides a framework within which the student can validate thinking. The use of nursing diagnosis without critical thinking is of no value to the nurse because, again, it becomes a rote process. Critical thinking is essential for accuracy of the diagnosis, and effective nursing actions are dependent upon this process. This question uses the same situation as above, with a different question asked of the student.

The 74-year-old client is admitted to PACU following an abdominal procedure under general anesthesia. He moans with pain and the nurse administers an opioid analgesic. One hour later, the client's vital signs are BP 104/62, P 54, R 11. He is receiving O_2 at 32% venti mask. ABG results are pH 7.28, PCO_2 55, PO_2 100, HCO_3 26. Which nursing diagnosis is most appropriate?

A) Impaired gas exchange

B) Ineffective airway clearance

C) Ineffective breathing patterns

D) Risk for aspiration

The student must apply age-related data (an elderly person receiving anesthesia), knowledge of the action of anesthesia and analgesics, interpretation of arterial blood gases, and knowledge of the distinguishing characteristics of the stated nursing diagnoses. To determine the best answer, the student must consider the respiratory rate and CO_2 retention as the priority diagnostic data.

31. Now the critical thinking exams are written, so I can relax, can't I?

Not hardly. It is amazing the amount of hard work entailed in writing, reviewing, updating, and revising questions. It is a never-ending process. A collection of good statistical evidence can be invaluable in test construction, but even an excellent question can show evidence over time of decreasing validity, as students become "wise" to the question. All test questions should be rotated, especially if a course is offered each semester. A substantial portion of questions should not be used in the subsequent semester, or even in the subsequent year. Additionally, new treatment approaches and nursing approaches are continually being developed and should be reflected in testing. So the process of developing a valid test bank is ongoing, but it does get easier over time, as quality items are developed.

The reward for all this work is seeing students be successful on NCLEX exams, making transitions to new specialty areas, and working in different facilities as safe and effective nurses in practice.

RESOURCES

McDonald, M. E. (2002). *Systematic assessment of learning outcomes: Developing multiple-choice exams.* Boston: Jones and Bartlett.

Morrison, S., Smith, P., & Britt, R. (1996). *Critical thinking and test item writing.* Livingston, TX: Century II Printing.

NCLEX-RN Test Plan. (2000). Retrieved May 20, 2002, from **http://www.ncsbn.org/**

Oermann, M. H., & Gaberson, K. B. (1998). *Evaluation and testing in nursing education.* New York: Springer.

Paul, R. (1998, April). *Critical thinking in nursing.* [Workshop]. Dallas, TX.

Recker, D. (2001). Postoperative respiratory status of a 76-year-old man. In M. Lunney (Ed.), *Critical thinking and nursing diagnosis: Case studies and analyses* (pp.132–135). Philadelphia: North American Nursing Diagnosis Association.

Chapter 8: Novice Nurse Learning Experiences

> *"... shall I teach you what knowledge is? When you know a thing, to recognize that you know it, and when you do not know a thing, to recognize that you do not know it. That is knowledge."*
>
> —Confucius

1. Why is critical thinking an essential component of helping novices in the profession become "good nurses" without loss of individuality?

Critical thinking as a process is the motivation for the evaluation question, "How effective is this nurse's clinical judgment?" Without an emphasis on critical thinking, other professional role aspects such as caring, communication, autonomy, and work style lack focus. Nurses at all levels are "works in progress" since the profession aims at continual improvement of its practitioners. Need for support and guidance is most evident when working with novice nurses, particularly student nurses and new graduates. Mentors of these novice nurses, including staff preceptors, clinical faculty, and other nurses, need both high quality presence and an awareness of their own strengths in critical thinking. Experienced nurses are able to make advanced judgments, but not always able to put into words how they "know what they know" in clinical decision making. Taking time to discern and verbalize their own clinical reasoning style can assist mentors to better guide novice nurses to be self aware in decision making regarding nursing care. One way to encourage novice nurses to put forth their own ideas is to ask them for their opinions on how a particular situation might be approached. Then mentors as experienced nurses can discuss other alternatives.

2. What are possible pitfalls of using critical thinking as a primary focus in assisting novice nurses in their professional development?

A strong emphasis on the conscious processes of critical thinking and their application by inexperienced nurses in clinical situations can be tedious and tiring. Unusual or extraneous data can assume exaggerated importance in otherwise routine situations of clinical care. Conscientious novices who want to show good judgment are particularly prone to "look for zebras" even when thinking symbolized by domestic animals would be more appropriate. Mentors of clinical novices in all fields of healthcare practitioner preparation have often used this classical metaphor by saying, "In ordinary situations, when you hear the pounding of hooves, the animal involved is more likely to be a horse than a zebra." The problem of overdoing analysis can be prevented by supporting inexperienced nurses in acquiring a thorough knowledge of frequently occurring patterns in patient care. I like to ask, "What is the most likely conclusion here?" Sometimes I call this the "Red Truck" approach. Walking to a nearby window, I point to a car or truck and ask, "If the driver of that vehicle were a close relative of this patient, what do you think that loved one would most worry about happening to the patient?" Once the baseline ideas are established in lay terms, then possibilities of more complex or unusual situations can be discussed.

3. Is critical thinking an adequate substitute for the use of the nursing process in assisting novice nurses to develop effective clinical judgment?

Any organized mode of thinking and responding can assist nurses to focus on important aspects of care. The nursing process when used alone has the danger of being too linear in its style, particularly in repetitive assignments such as written nursing care plans. Too strong an overlap with the medical model is an even more traditional style of responding and can lead to nurse passivity because of mainly dependent nursing behaviors. Critical thinking, like elementary scientific methods, can be used too generally as a vague approach to logical thinking, leading to a tendency to "shoot an arrow into the air and wherever it lands call it the target"—a version of foggy reasoning.

Beginning nurses are novices at detecting dangers of an inadequate conceptual map to support practice. Any frame of reference when used alone, even by experienced clinicians, has the possibility of leading with its weaknesses. Perhaps the best approach with inexperienced nurses is to combine the nursing process with critical thinking methods such as concept maps, focused questioning, and selected creative problem solving approaches.

4. What two main critical thinking areas form the basis for all goals, placements, assignments, supervision, and evaluation of clinical learning experiences for those who are learning how to be effective nurses?

The two themes involved in all nursing clinical experience are:

- Patient-centered nursing care
- Professional role development

The two themes basically involve these introspective questions:

Am I doing the right thing with and for this individual patient?

How does this behavior fit into the role of the professional nurse?

The promotion of effective and aware nursing care requires good outcome-based planning. Designing such focused objectives begins with "What do I want end results to be?" We also use formal guidelines such as the American Nurses Association clinical standards for general and specialty nursing care to be clear on what we expect of a "good nurse." Only then do we move into the priority skills required and the knowledge that supports those skills. These interrelated steps help to sort "need to know" versus "nice to know" or the whimsical "nuts to know" categories of learning experiences.

I have used the following methods for assisting new nurses with professional role development:

- Be clear regarding specific desired observable areas of competency.
- State in plain, understandable terms the "why" of these competencies. Cite some actual positive outcomes or "success stories" observed in the clinical area.
- Sometimes it also helps to give examples of the "negative case" of what happens when the nursing care does *not* meet acceptable standards.
- Involve new nurses in discussions on professional values and how to incorporate them into daily care.
- Use some meaningful self-assessment guides that will help novice nurses answer, "How am I doing as a professional nurse?"

The examination of how well novice nurses are performing in their care and how well they are developing as individual nurses is less threatening if other nurses are being asked the same question. There is more "ownership" of standards when it is obvious that they are really valued in a clinical area and are not just for the "new kids on the block."

5. What types of critical thinking in professional role behaviors should novice nurses demonstrate at various progression levels?

The areas of role behaviors expected of student nurses and new graduates in their progression toward full professional nurse job-readiness include communication, teamwork, autonomy, active engagement in learning, and self-awareness in role development (see Table 8.1).

6. What types of clinical supervision promote critical thinking by novice nurses?

In order to avoid a "Guess what I am thinking" approach to supervision, teachers and preceptors who guide the learning of new nurses need to be

TABLE 8.1 Role Behaviors and Development

Role Component	Role Characteristics
Communication Level:	
The wording we use indicates specific levels of knowledge and judgment.	
We need to use wording that is compatible with our ability.	
Beginner: the basic "who, what, when, where" questions	**Beginner:** Sometimes we are unfamiliar with certain concepts or equipment and come across as a "beginner" in that area. At early levels in their clinical education or in a new area, learners ask a lot of "beginner" questions such as what they should do first or where equipment is located. Although all practicing nurses have some occasions to use elementary questions, developing nurses are expected to change the level and style of their primary communication as they move to more advanced levels of knowledge and skills.
Advanced: "I see that you are using your PCA every ten minutes. Are you getting enough pain relief or are you still in pain?"	**Advanced:** Validating or verifying questions involves verbalization of what is already known about a situation or observation, followed by an impression about those apparent facts, and then a question on the areas of doubt or knowledge deficit on the topic addressed. This focused communication approach is often used by experienced nurses seeking peer consultation. It gives an impression that the questioner is "on board" with the current situation but wants support in further critical thinking and decision making.
Expert: "In my years as a geriatric psych specialist, I have seen the urgent need to carefully monitor medication dosing in older patients."	**Expert:** Occasionally we communicate as experts who do not need extensive verification of information with colleagues. This is very rare and can create the suspicion of hiding lack of ability if used inappropriately.

TABLE 8.1   Role Behaviors and Development *(continued)*

Role Component	Role Characteristics
Communication Focus:	
Area of main concern	Some novice nurses are slow to get to the point on priority topics due either to lack of knowledge or lack of communication ability. Others at more advanced levels may feel pressure to over-verbalize to show assessment skills. All nurses can profit from using a "newspaper" approach for conveying clinical information. Front Page: Use for priority topics. Get to the point immediately. State the topic of concern in the first one to three sentences. Back Pages: Use for less important data. Here a more conversational style with less focus delays the main point. This is more like a newspaper's later sections, such as commentaries on political, social, or sports topics.
Communication Content:	
Data	**What to say:** Content of clinical reporting should include statements of obviously important data plus impressions of patient health status and response to care.
When to share data	**Timing:** The reporting of vital information should be done as soon as it is detected so that "yellow flag" data can motivate quick action before "red flag" crises emerge. The best time to report a suspected deviation from the expected is as early as possible. **Routines:** Regular patterns of checking in with faculty or staff mentors need to be established, including pre-conference planning, mid-shift consultation, and end-of-shift summaries.

TABLE 8.1 Role Behaviors and Development *(continued)*

Role Component	Role Characteristics
Communication Content:	
Importance	**Recording:** Effective documentation maintains quality control in relation to professional, ethical, and legal standards.
Teamwork:	
Peer and staff support	**Aim:** A community of caring. A focus on assigned learning and practice experiences is essential, but novice nurses are also expected to participate with other nurses in mutual tasks related to patient care, supplies, task support, and reporting.
Identification of behaviors for positive team development—Critical thinking and learning regarding team functioning includes feedback on team participation styles.	**Acknowledgment:** To build team loyalty. Some personal interaction styles lend themselves easily to teamwork but need to be acknowledged by mentors on how they specifically contribute to team functioning. More reserved individuals can be complimented on their respect for others and also given strategies to actively share their ideas and energy with other team members.
Autonomy:	
Grounded self-direction	**Clear meaning:** New nurses often need clarification of what autonomy involves. It is a demonstration of good judgment and the ability to make decisions. Novices may believe that being a nurse means never having to check in with peers or supervisors.
Balance of dependence, interdependence, and autonomy	**Balance:** Inexperienced nurses may swing between extremes of dependence and independence in their clinical functioning. Those who are overly cautious need assistance in thinking through how to use their strengths in more assertive ways. Action-oriented, independent individuals who are highly self-directed may believe that keeping others informed would show deficits in

TABLE 8.1   Role Behaviors and Development *(continued)*

Role Component	Role Characteristics
Autonomy:	
Balance of dependence, interdependence, and autonomy *(continued)*	knowledge, judgment, or skills. Critical thinking consultations by education faculty and staff preceptors can empower developing nurses to gain the balance of real autonomy, which includes a verifying style of communication, reporting, and peer consultation.
Clinical Presence:	
Engagement in the situation at hand	A trusting partnership atmosphere in the clinical area can promote a free exchange of ideas and help new nurses be willing to participate fully in the professional role. To increase engagement in critical thinking about aspects of the professional nurse role, mentors can verbalize why certain role behaviors are important.
Persistence: Staying long enough to appreciate the "big picture"	Nurses are involved with both depth and scope of clinical challenges. Novice nurses may miss the depth of judgment necessary in care if they detach attention after brief observation experiences, become bored, and ask permission to move on to other assignments or placements. Mentors can share the scope of care by discussing factors in the "big picture" such as family, professional, accreditation, financial, legal, and public "stakeholder" issues in effective and efficient nursing care.
Role Self-Awareness:	
Individual development	Students and new graduates can be encouraged to compare their styles of decision making and nursing care with those of others. They need to state clear goals for professional development in routine verbal exchanges, in clinical journals, and in periodic evaluations with mentors. Each novice nurse needs guidance in

TABLE 8.1 Role Behaviors and Development *(continued)*

Role Component	Role Characteristics
Role Self-Awareness:	
Individual development *(continued)* Working toward a personal philosophy Crafting own practice to be consistent with values	developing a personal philosophy of nursing and a career mission statement. Progress in the development of role strengths or a reduction in role deficits should be acknowledged by teachers and preceptors.

very specific. Like the sign in shopping malls with an arrow and note saying, "You are here," individuals in learning situations need directional reminders.

Here are some "roadmap" indicators that can keep everyone moving toward effective care behaviors:

- **Shared standards.** Agreement on clear standards and on how critical thinking will be measured in evaluation needs to be established early in the orientation period.
- **Partnership promotion.** Active engagement of faculty or staff mentors with students and new graduates is essential in the development of clinical reasoning. In education and management vocabulary, we speak of "building community" with one another.
- **Reflective strategies.** Some of the supervision techniques that are most effective in promoting critical thinking are focused questioning, guided reasoning, and exercises in creative thinking.
- **Concurrent feedback.** Evaluation of critical incidents can occur through shared on-site experiences, clinical journals, and critical incident analyses in individual and group clinical conferences. As for when to schedule such feedback, the best answer is "As close to the triggering event as possible."
- **"Walking the talk."** Role modeling by mentors gives opportunities to demonstrate how standards are applied to nursing situations as well as to explore decision-making styles. Mentors are especially encouraged to verbalize their reasoning concurrently with their actions so that students gain insight as well as critical thinking vocabulary. I have often referred to this as a type of "newscasting" in which descriptions are verbalized in the middle of the action scene.

7. How can critical thinking processes be used to help student nurses and new graduates make the transition to the role of the professional nurse from other more familiar helping behaviors?

The similarity of nursing to other helping roles such as friend, family member, or neighbor can be used as a point of departure to introduce the more specialized purpose and behaviors of a professional nurse. Layperson helping roles are limited at times to keeping a respectful distance from the person being helped. Novice nurses may not see that a professional helping role involves behaviors such as asking rather personal questions and doing frequent physical examinations. Critical thinking processes assist these nurses in "bridging" theoretical knowledge with the desire to help other human beings using nursing skills.

I like to first acknowledge what aspects of lay caring a student or inexperienced nurse is using. I might comment, "I see you are showing respect for the patient's privacy by not asking about sensitive matters right away." Then we can go on to discuss how nurses can build on basic rapport to gather and use information for patient care. Mentors can show how more advanced communication and action can help individuals in ways which are far more complex and significant than what family or friends can do. Here are some examples of ways to promote more advanced caring:

- Role modeling on how to move from superficial topics to focused interviewing on reasons the patient is seeking help.
- Focused patient questions such as, "How does this pain episode compare to what you have experienced in the past?"
- Use of case studies that illustrate nurse assessment and decision making.
- Practice on phrases to use in introducing the nurse's role, such as, "As part of my job, I need to ask you..." Novice nurses can also practice ways to help patients make the transition into more therapeutic communication. For example, they can give patients thoughtful descriptions of why physical examinations and procedures are being done.
- Guided analysis of the patient care record with questions such as, "Why do you think the healthcare team has this particular plan of care for this individual?"
- Discussions before and after procedures to help novice nurses connect technical aspects of care with theoretical knowledge. (We sabotage this aim if we do too much quizzing in the middle of procedures. Psychomotor skills require concentration without a lot of interruption.)

Inexperienced nurses need help in combining effective aspects of care with more detached reasoning and principles. Without such links, novices draw on more casual ways such as social conversation and vague reassurance to relate to patients. These reflective bridges can help new nurses give truly holistic care by using their own abilities in a holistic way. Otherwise role functions are divided into separate areas using head or heart or hands. Nurses then become theoretical experts whose helping applications are technical and superficial.

8. What focused questioning approaches by clinical faculty and preceptors can best demonstrate effective levels of critical thinking regarding patient-centered nursing care?

Questioning of novice nurses by mentors in the clinical area can be anticipatory (rehearsing before a particular situation), concurrent with clinical activities or mentor role modeling, or as a follow-up critical analysis to clarify priorities. The areas of questioning listed in Table 8.2 are consistent with steps of the nursing process but are not limited to the usual sequence of that process.

9. How can critical thinking for effective priority setting be learned in busy acute care settings where multitasking by staff nurses appears chaotic?

A busy acute care nursing unit often looks like a crowded anthill teeming with a level of action which appears to have no detectable order. Like the anthill, a closer examination reveals a high degree of systematized organization and task specialization. Individual nurses are simultaneously accomplishing multiple complex tasks in high tech, high data, high stress situations. They are able to quickly adapt to rapid changes and concentrate on deciding what they should do, think, or feel in responding to healthcare needs of individuals.

Guided rehearsals for novice nurses and student nurses prior to entering busy care units can help them detect ways order is somehow maintained in such settings. Here are some ways to accomplish preparation through "risk projection" practice:

1. **Group or Individual Role Play Conferences.** Realistic scenarios are given, followed by questions such as, "How would you handle this?" or "What will you do if this happens?" or "What would be the nurse's most effective response?"

2. **Shadowing.** Each newcomer can be assigned to stay with one nurse for a period of time and then list observations of judgment situations.

3. **Teamwork.** A new nurse can also be asked to document or "track" how each nurse's actions contribute to teamwork in complex team situations.

4. **Group Role Division.** Classical group roles such as organizer or motivator can be explored in post-observation clinical conferences. Novices are cued

TABLE 8.2 Focused Questioning Approaches

Question/Focus	Strategies	Strategic Rationale
Who?		
Specifics on patients: Individuals and groups	• Determine the most likely response. • Tailor action to the patient, situation, and resources.	Novice nurses need to be able to identify the two to three "standard" nursing responses for a particular type of clinical situation and to describe expected evidence-based outcomes. Nursing actions with and for patients are also individualized and tailored to all aspects of the person's health status and health values. Available resources are also considered.
What and why?		
Patient assessment and focused chart review The "why" of data assessment involves a continual referencing to clinical principles from texts or experts so that reasoning and judgment are grounded in accepted bodies of knowledge.	• Which patient to see first • What to do first in routine and emergency situations • How often to repeat basic or specialized assessments	Questioning and role modeling by clinical mentors can foster understanding of the decision-making process related to timing of nurse behaviors. Experienced clinicians are able to quickly decide timing issues in planning care. Individuals with infection control alerts, one whose pain level is not responding to large or frequent doses of analgesics, or someone whose vital signs show erratic or disturbing patterns take priority in time organization.
So what?		
Bottom line implications	Judgment assistance and role modeling on: • When to collaborate • To whom referral is appropriate • What data to have ready when contact is made	Health care is collaborative and is also often very time pressured for all providers. Both routine and urgent nursing responsibilities must fit into a busy schedule. Experts we consult ask that we "get to the bottom line" as quickly as possible. To do good referrals, good critical thinking and focused communication are skills needed by nurses at all clinical levels.

TABLE 8.2 Focused Questioning Approaches *(continued)*

Question/Focus	Strategies	Strategic Rationale
Now what?		
Priority actions	• Interview patient. • Assess patient record. • Study trends.	What personal data such as gender, age, developmental stage, and subjective account of life events can give clues as to actual or specific patient needs?
When?		

Timing/ sequence of nurse actions	• Data collection:
	  General and focused
	• Data comparison:
	  Compare data against expected or "classical" patterns regarding health status, signs and symptoms, treatments, medications, and patient response to interventions.
	• Data reporting:
	  Reporting of data that do not seem to fit the expected or usual picture can help solve apparent "mysteries" and model ways to detect the need for further data.
		Initial assessment often involves a quick general assessment of overall functioning and then more intense focus on data relevant to known or probable main problems.
		
		These focused data are combined with later, more thorough assessments, health record data such as diagnostic test results, and reports of other healthcare providers.
		
		An unusual laboratory examination result, the ordering of an extremely strong or experimental medication, prolonged treatment beyond the usual regimen for similar conditions, or even statements by patients, families, or healthcare providers that things do not "seem right" are all potential reasons to do further assessment.

What before?		
Preparation for collaboration	• Prioritize three to five main concerns. • Propose a best hope and worst fear. • Compare expected with unusual data and draw conclusions on planning and implementation.	Experienced clinicians think in clusters of important data and can zero in on relevant data, such as regard to individuals with severe infections, those on immune suppressive therapies, and early clues of complications such as sepsis, organ failure, or psychological withdrawal from participation in recommended treatment plans.

beforehand to look for roles with questions such as, "Who is really in charge?" "Who furnishes information?" "Who is a good motivator?"

5. **The Big Team Picture.** Orientation of inexperienced nurses and students can begin with very specific task assignments combined with open-ended exploration of all the caregivers involved in specific patient situations. For example, each new nurse chooses a particular patient. Then I ask, "What other health team members in and out of this department will be involved in the plan of care for this patient?" Each nurse can "follow" the route taken by a real or fictitious patient from intake through admissions and special care-giver interventions.

10. How can inexperienced nurses be taught to stay alert and use critical thinking in more tranquil settings or on quiet days in usually highly active areas?

Quiet, evenly paced nursing care environments are more common in community-based settings and yet they also occur at intervals in acute care and even critical care areas. Sometimes student nurses and new graduates are misled by the apparent calm of care situations or the ability of individual nurses to never appear to lose their air of tranquility. These novice observers draw conclusions that nothing of interest or concern is happening. They can be lulled into complacency or boredom, both of which take the edge off critical thinking abilities.

The impression inexperienced nurses get of a quiet situation is that of a tranquil picture with no disturbances, like that of a duck smoothly swimming across a quiet lake. What they do not know is that beneath the calm surface the duck is paddling like crazy. Experienced nurses, especially those in leadership positions, have continuous internal dialogues in which data are processed, problems identified, and focused planning done.

Here is a typical internal dialogue involving an experienced nurse in an acute care setting:

> "We will probably have lots of discharges and new admissions today, so everyone will be busy. We probably ought to assign a couple of people to the two patients who required a lot of care yesterday. Then the rest of us can divide the discharge and admitting tasks so all the bases are covered."

One way to help novice nurses maintain quality judgment in situations with variable or low-key activity levels is to build clinical assignments around focused clinical objectives that define "mastery skills," which must each be completed, but with flexible timelines. Such skills delineate critical behaviors that capture key concepts in important areas of clinical nursing. Statements of mastery skills give categories of important role behaviors, along with a list of sample ways to meet the requirement.

Sample mastery skill: Demonstrate awareness of safety measures for older patients.

Ways to complete this requirement:

1. Plan and implement safety teaching for one older patient.
2. Explain a relevant nursing journal article on geriatric safety risks.
3. Take a quiz on agency safety policies regarding care of older adults.

11. What is an "All Points Bulletin" approach to clinical documentation and how can it help inexperienced nurses become more focused in their charting?

Police and security agents become immediately alert when an All Points Bulletin or "APB" is broadcast. Another type of APB, representing Alive, Problem, and Body Systems, can be used to focus novice nurse observations, reporting, and documentation. These four areas (including safety) of priority assessment need attention several times a day in an acute care setting. Overall, assessment documentation needs to follow five essential rules, including Clarity, Focus, Data Support, Concerns, and No Mysteries.

- **Alive** means to note the precise level of consciousness and activity along with cardio-respiratory vital signs. An example would be for the nurse to state not merely that the patient is "awake" but more precisely whether the individual is responsive, answers questions appropriately, and is participating in nursing care. Sometimes to justify a vague assessment of level of consciousness, a novice will state, "His eyes were open." The recording of heart and respiratory status needs to include numbers as well as quality of each along with readings from any special monitors in place. Such data should always be included in a focused assessment, even if the situation remains stable. Baseline data are the latest recorded observation and not just the first charting of the day.

- **Problem** indicates data related to the main physical or non-physical (emotional, sociocultural, developmental, spiritual, health teaching) reason the individual is seeking or receiving healthcare. The current health challenge may involve one specific problem or a cluster of related health challenges. If the setting or situation has more of a focus on health promotion or disease prevention, then "Problem" may mean the topic requiring the most substantial attention. If the problem is physical, then assessment involves observations and questions on major related body systems, the presence and status of procedures such as intravenous fluids or gastric suction, and the individual's response to nursing care related to the problem.

"Episodic and emergency" observations and documentation indicate changes in the patient's condition, location, or caregiving team, and may certainly be related to a problem category.

- **Body Systems** are data ranging from an initial cursory examination to a full head-to-toe assessment. Either category needs to include a strong emphasis on gastrointestinal and renal functioning. Specifics should include tolerance of food and fluids, with exact amounts compared to individualized goals such as life-sustaining calorie estimations and expected hydration needs for age and condition. A check of gastrointestinal functioning requires more than a check for bowel sounds along with Yes or No questioning on whether there has been a bowel movement that day. Every day nurses need to ask the time of the last bowel movement and describe its quality, from nurse observations or the individual or family account. Day eight in the care of anyone is no time to be surprised the person has had no bowel function other than bowel sounds. A check of renal functioning also needs to be precise, including frequency of urination, estimated or measured amounts, and any related symptoms. Persons with a history of renal malfunction also need to be checked for special dietary restrictions such as limited fluid or protein, their tolerance of these limitations, and signs of complications such as fluid retention. Details about other body systems need to be noted as appropriate. Novices should be cautioned not to elaborate extensively in reporting or recording about non-problem systems lest they unnecessarily raise "red-flag" suspicions among other nurses.

- **Safety** is the fourth major assessment category added when a plural "S" is added to the APB reminder system. Safety equipment such as bedside rails needs to be noted, along with any special safety help needed, such as "Assisted to the bathroom."

12. How can a mentor for inexperienced nurses assist them to include non-physical data in assessments?

Novice nurses tend to be at extreme points of the spectrum, either making non-physical data the primary focus of assessment or ignoring them. For those who tend to omit this important area of observation and care, this focused sentence completion assignment may help.

Emotional Empathy: Ask the new staff nurse or student nurse to "guess" what an individual (even an infant or unconscious child or adult) may be feeling and thinking in the current situation by completing these sentences *without* interviewing the person.

I feel . . .

I am afraid that . . .

I hope . . .

My care has been . . .

People here are . . .

My family and friends . . .

Probably what will happen to me . . .

Developmental Awareness:

My main role in life recently has been . . .

I am considered at the developmental stage of . . .

Ways you can tell I am at this stage are . . .

Ways my current health affects my role include . . .

My best role hope right now is . . .

My worst role fear is that . . .

Sociocultural Context:

My place in the family and community is . . .

My family believes that health and illness are . . .

The type of care we traditionally expect is . . .

The staff needs to consider that we . . .

My current support system is . . .

Mentors can assist in analyzing the hypothetical answers given, not only to check insight into the patient's actual situation, but also to ascertain the nurse's style of answering. Both approaches can give mentors appraisal data to assist the development of the staff or student nurse in non-physical assessment and care.

13. What elements of interviewing skills do novice nurses need in order to discern how a current illness or health experience fits into an individual's overall health pattern?

Individuals with long term problems such as chronic physical or mental illness especially need nurses to understand their current situations in a larger context. Novice nurses can gain skill in this type of contextual perspective by using

TABLE 8.3 Interview Questions

Area of concern	Nurse exploration of topic
Early problem	"How did you first realize that you might have a problem in this area?"
Diagnosis	"What kind of difficulties did you have in finding out what was wrong?"
Patterns	"Tell me how the problem has changed or stayed the same over time."
Response to care	"What was it like for you and your family to go through all this?
Adjustment	"In what ways have you had to adjust your goals and daily activities because of this situation?"

focused interviewing techniques. Open-ended questions give patients opportunities to explain their "stories" in a personal way (see Table 8.3).

Inexperienced nurses such as students and new graduates may need coaching and rehearsal in keeping questions open-ended, waiting for answers, probing for more detail, clarifying inconsistent data, and being empathetic toward the individuals and families facing long term challenges.

14. What is the value of assigning a critical analysis of patient health records?

Experienced nurse clinicians, even nursing faculty and experienced nursing staff preceptors, often assume that novice nurses can quickly zero in on key information in patient health records. (I have found that some experienced nurses cannot do this as well, and benefit from the demonstration below. When they tell me they do "not have time to read the chart," that is a pretty good clue that they are not really familiar with the process of assessing a chart systematically.) Once the elements of patients' charts are introduced and variations in specialty records pointed out, the matter of how to assess a record is considered a given. Clinical beginners waste time doing leisurely front to back reading of charts, copying all lab reports, and getting distracted with peripheral data. They can be assisted to go directly to the skeletal outline of a written record. This bare-bones core includes relevant personal and home data, major history and physical problems, reason for current healthcare intervention, and results of classic diagnostic tests for major problems.

Demonstration by an "expert." As experienced clinicians, faculty and staff mentors can role model a focused records analysis with a three to five minute demonstration. During the analysis, the clinician needs to verbalize verification of expected data, clues to why certain goals are used for treatment and care, and identified "mysteries" still needing to be solved. The following points give a partial picture of such a demonstration:

- **Core data first.** Go directly to the intake summary or admission notes and examine these questions together: Why did this person come for healthcare assistance? What has this person's general health been like overall in the past? What seem to be the patient's main strengths and current health challenges? Describe the individual's personal support system.

- **Diagnostic data.** What tests have been ordered and why? What impressions do you get of the results?

- **Progress summaries.** Scan all health team entries on what has happened since admission to the healthcare system. In a lengthy record, read the latest entry first, then read only the "Impressions" sections of the other entries. (The rest can be read in detail later.)

- **Ask.** What is going on? What are the current conclusions about this patient's condition, progress, and prognosis?

- **Conclusions.** State the three main concerns affecting nursing care for this patient and family.

An appropriate baseline expectation is that the new caregivers will do daily critical chart review for all patients to whom they are assigned. In addition, other charts with critical incident potential should be checked, and at least a few random "chart audits" should be done using agency forms for quality assurance documentation experience. This is a good practice for all nurses.

15. How can computer-assisted instruction (CAI) programs promote critical thinking?

One advantage of electronic media in clinical instruction is that learners can access CAI programs in a computer laboratory, a health library or media site, and often from a home computer. Self-paced completion of nursing content and processes on clinical topics can supplement classroom and clinical learning, meet individual information needs, and remediate identified gaps in clinical performance. However, computer-assisted programs can be "busy work" if they do not specifically fit into focused learning objectives. Baseline requirements can be made across course or orientation groups in regard to required numbers and types of software programs to be completed. A continuing education format may be used with pre- and post-tests to check related knowledge, even if continuing education credit is not given. In addition, individuals with inadequate performance on written theory or clinical tests, clinical mastery skills, or standardized testing on nursing topics may be required to complete additional programs focused on content and process deficits.

Sample CAI assignment: Together the mentor and novice nurse identify "gaps" in previous learning or performance. This can be done through self-assessment approaches, mentor observations, or written tests. Then a specific assignment can be made. For example, a new nurse or student with very little postoperative recovery care experience can be assigned to view a CAI program on this topic and then furnish a list of five possible complications.

16. How can educator and preceptor evaluation of novice nurse critical thinking be made a more positive experience for everyone involved?

Evaluation of applied critical thinking can be concurrently integrated with other clinical experiences rather than saved as the "last step" in a linear process. Ongoing evaluation works best in an atmosphere of trust and positive mutual goals. Actual or simulated clinical problems can be approached as a team, with learning potential for novices as well as mentors. Questioning on clinical topics can include encouragement to give a "best guess" along with supportive information believed to be true.

First, I can establish trust by saying, "Let's each give two things we think are fairly obvious in this situation." Then I might go on to ask the novice nurse, "What is your hunch on what might happen next to this patient? What gave you clues to this impression?" Responses are best expressed in a comprehensive but down-to-earth manner. An over-emphasis on critical thinking and a specialized vocabulary can inadvertently inhibit active participation in verbalizing plans and self-evaluation. Novices need to know that it really is okay to verbalize commonly accepted information, what I call "stating the obvious." For example, if a new nurse starts to explain effects of a commonly administered medication by citing very rare complications, the preceptor can say, "Let's back up to the basics first. What are the effects that you have known about for a long time and which will *not* be on the evening news? They are so common that the patient probably already knows about them." Once basics are established, the new or rare information brought by the student nurse or new employee can be acknowledged, assessed, and perhaps shared with others.

Positive questioning and collaboration, immediate feedback, alternative answers, acknowledgment of strengths, and trusting intuition can all be integrated into sound evaluation combining trust with focused principles of critical thinking.

17. How can nursing faculty and staff preceptors use critical thinking to detect and balance the "gifts" novice nurses demonstrate in particular aspects of nursing care?

Inexperienced individuals learning the nursing role combine thinking and learning styles with personal tendencies and preferences in deciding what part of nursing care they routinely emphasize. Often the chosen area of emphasis is acknowledged by others as a strength and can become that person's most comfortable mode of responding. Examples are those who are particularly good at attention to detail in data gathering (and love to chart it!), those who are especially attentive to the psychosocial needs of patients (and spend lots of time talking to the patients), and those who show initiative in seeking new experiences (possibly helping to insert that chest tube even when they should be medicating the patient to whom they are assigned).

Any area of strength can become a deficiency if it is overused or not balanced by other abilities. Sometimes, observers such as clinical faculty or agency staff detect deficits in overall novice nurse performance and conclude that a "gift" such as constant data gathering is actually a negative behavior. Mentors can take time to pause and find the special ability behind a negative behavior. Then a misused "gift" can be redirected so new nurses can build on actual strengths and try more comprehensive approaches. Someone who is obsessed with assessment can be encouraged to get to the bottom line on priority data and then move on to planning and implementation of nursing care. High-energy individuals who want to jump into action without adequate assessment or planning can be acknowledged for their efficiency and encouraged to slow down and think through situations carefully.

All this detection and balancing of gifts is best facilitated by clinical faculty and staff mentors who are aware of their *own* caregiving styles as well as ways to empower novice nurses in development of a sound repertoire of responses to patient needs.

18. How can a coaching agreement between student nurses and faculty or staff mentors be used to focus critical thinking in clinical experiences?

The process of coaching can be used as an "upfront" planning method and is also valuable for early intervention on possible performance problems. During student or employee orientations to a new clinical area, coaching can be used to make agreements on performance goals. Sometimes these are called "contracts" but it is good to check the novice nurse's impression of the term since some schools and agencies use contracting for self-paced learning and others reserve it for possible "red-flag" signs of safety issues.

Coaching used in planning new learning, orientation, or refresher experiences often involves a reward system of some sort. This might take the form of special recognition for good performance, tailoring learning or orientation goals to fit individual preferences, or the option of omitting or redesigning certain requirements. For example, novices who are doing well in assessing care and identifying both the obvious and the less obvious patient needs may be allowed the opportunity to work with the patients in the disease category they are most interested in and want to pursue, such as patients with diabetes.

As soon as borderline problems are detected with critical thinking in the clinical area, a focused coaching conference can be scheduled. I often promote agreement by saying, "We need to clarify some things about your performance. Let's work together to get you on track and head off any possible problems 'at the pass.'" At an agreed upon time, we then work together to complete performance flowcharts or checklists such as the one by Fournies (2000) or the one by Mager and Pipe (1996). The conference always starts with a summary of any strengths the novice nurse has demonstrated. This is followed with a discussion on possible performance deficits, a topic introduced by exploring, "Is there a problem here?" Questioning or the use of accountability flow charts can be used to arrive at an agreement on what the specific problem is, whether changes are advised, and if further training in knowledge or skills is indicated. Then remediation plans are made to improve the situation using resources such as nursing texts and journals, consultation with experts, computer-assisted learning aids, or referenced writing assignments to demonstrate knowledge of critical thinking principles related to the identified clinical deficit. The written coaching agreement needs to document data on the clinical problem, describe the coaching procedure, list recommended resources, assign activities and written work, then end with timelines and signatures of the mentor and the nurse being coached. Follow-up sessions are scheduled for feedback on progress. If the clinical deficit does not improve to a satisfactory level, stronger measures such as an administrative contract, clinical incident report, or clinical probation may be necessary.

19. What is the best timing for teacher or mentor intervention when severe critical thinking deficits become apparent?

The best timing is an immediate response, as close to incidents of demonstrated problems as possible. If patient safety is involved in critical thinking and clinical performance deficits, the pace is that of crisis intervention. Often the student or new graduate involved is withdrawn from the clinical area until facts can be established. At times, alternate assignments are appropriate so that clinical hours can continue to be meaningfully accumulated in case remediation and resumption of regularly scheduled clinical experiences are possible.

With more subtle and cumulative evidence of performance problems over several days or multiple assigned activities, the minimum timing for initial major conferencing is at least by the mid-point of the clinical rotation or orientation period. The final evaluation conference or even the last week of a scheduled clinical experience cannot meet criteria for optimal timing of important evaluation feedback. The most positive and least threatening system involves an early sharing of planned "checkpoint" dates. I like to use simple self-assessment tools as "tickets" to these mini-conferences so that we start with the novice nurse's own impressions of how things are going.

For both gradual and sudden problems, documentation of observed behaviors by faculty and staff mentors is urgent and needs to be concurrently shared with the involved individual when possible. The objective of a "no surprises" approach to evaluation is to naturally integrate mentor feedback, both positive and negative, into other aspects of professional development. When combined with frequent verbal feedback, including compliments for progress on challenging areas, the novice nurse's problems with critical thinking can often be remedied. I actually have seen early intervention to "head off" a borderline problem empower the novice nurse with the problem to "leap frog" and surpass peer performance. Much of this positive potential in a negative situation can be attributed to how much ownership or "buy-in" can be secured through partnership efforts focused on examining possible solutions as a team. This is not the world against the novice, but rather an approach of supportive development, in which you are all willing to work together to improve this situation.

20. What can mentors say on performance appraisals of staff and student nurses to demonstrate "tracking" of critical thinking development?

Four areas of evaluation can use specific wording intended to describe critical thinking abilities in novice nurses. These areas are Standards, Behavioral Observations, Overall Performance, and Developmental Plan.

- The Standards category refers to specific concepts or documents used to measure nurse or student performance. For example, "This individual has shown special strength in the first of the agency mission goals which is…" or, "Ranking of performance in steps of the nursing process areas starting with the best area..." "Needs improvement in these two major skills which show effective care for patients recovering from major surgery ..."

- Behavioral Observations can give examples of documentation in various performance areas, such as teamwork judgment. "She often completes her work early and then decides where her help could best be used by other nurses." Isolated incidents, positive or negative, need to be cited as such and kept in context. For example, "He usually shows good judgment in room assignment of patients and is able to quickly correct inappropriate plans, such as when he rejected the proposal to place someone being admitted with an infection to a room with a post-operative patient."

- Overall Performance summarizes the use of clinical judgment. Critical thinking before, during, and after nursing care should be examined and relative strengths assessed. "Although this nurse is a bit hesitant in assessing complex or unusual situations, she is very efficient once she has verified her judgment on an appropriate plan." "Progress continues in analyzing how work could have been improved, such as during times of multiple patient admissions."

- Developmental Plan consists of goals mutually arrived at by the mentor/nurse team. Wording should show clear future demonstration of critical thinking related to performance and should also indicate verbalized agreements. "Her main stated goal is improvement of setting priorities so that major areas of patient needs are given more efficient and effective attention." "He has been instructed to view the following procedural videotapes and has agreed to submit his summary of how they can help his judgment in the problem area within the next two weeks."

RESOURCES

Benner, P., Hooper-Kyriakidis, P. H., & Stannard, D. (1999). *Clinical wisdom and interventions in critical care: A thinking-in-action approach.* Philadelphia: Saunders.

Evans, J. A. (1997). A holistic model for moving toward excellence in chaotic times. *The Journal of Continuing Education in Nursing, 28*(4), 157–163.

Facione, N. C., & Facione, P. A. (1996). Externalizing the critical thinking in knowledge development and clinical judgment. *Nursing Outlook, 44*(3), 129–136.

Fournies, F. F. (2000). *Coaching for improved work performance* (3rd ed.). Whitby, Ontario, Canada: McGraw Hill/Ryerson.

Grealish, L. (2000). The skills of coach are an essential element in clinical learning. *Journal of Nursing Education, 39*(5), 231–233.

Lee, J. E. M., & Ryan Wenger, N. (1997). The "Think Out Loud" seminar for teaching clinical reasoning: A case study of a child with pharyngitis. *Journal of Pediatric Health Care, 11*(3), 101–110.

Mager, R. F., & Pipe, P. (1996). *A quick reference checklist: For use in analyzing performance problems.* Atlanta: Center for Effective Performance.

Mattingly, C., & Fleming, M. H. (1994). *Clinical reasoning: Forms of inquiry in a therapeutic practice.* Philadelphia: F. A. Davis.

Paul, R. W., & Heaslip, P. (1995). Critical thinking and intuitive nursing practice. *Journal of Advanced Nursing, 22,* 40–47.

Chapter 9: Staff Perceptions and Effects

"The conventional view serves to protect us from the painful job of thinking."

—John Kenneth Galbraith, economist, Harvard professor, author

1. It seems like some nurses are focused more on tasks than on critical thinking. Is that a common finding around the country today?

Nurse managers and administrators report that many staff nurses, especially new graduates, are very task-oriented. But the performance of any task should be accompanied by critical thinking. As an example, take dressing changes; proper procedure requires thinking about the answers to these questions *before* the task is performed:

- Do I have the right treatment plan for the right patient?
- Why is the patient getting this dressing change?
- What assessments are required prior to changing the dressing?
- What else might I need to do prior to the dressing change?
- What adverse effects do I need to monitor for?
- What if adverse effects occur—what should I do?
- What changes might be necessary in the currently ordered process?
- Is there any teaching that needs to be done?
- What documentation is needed?

As you can see, there is more to changing a dressing than just gathering the supplies and forging ahead. In some cases, we change dressings that are not really needed, or that would be better changed more or less frequently. I have had the unfortunate experience of observing nurses attempt to change very painful dressings without pre-medicating the patient, and who have offered the excuse that there was not sufficient time to do so. This is definitely not critical thinking, but it clearly represents a task orientation.

2. Are some healthcare settings more likely to have task-oriented nurses than others?

Some healthcare settings lend themselves to being less task-focused and more outcome-oriented. In rehabilitation settings, for example, the entire healthcare team focuses on meeting client outcomes related to achieving independent function. All members of the team, including nurses, use critical thinking skills to plan and implement interventions that meet those identified, expected outcomes.

By contrast, acute care clients spend an average of just a few days in the hospital. The number of required tasks is usually higher in acute care when compared to rehabilitation and long-term care settings. As the nursing shortage increases, medical-surgical nurses are especially prone to being task directed. Most of these nurses are less experienced because they tend to leave the med-surg units once they have a year or two of experience. These units have become the "training ground" or "springboard" for transfer to specialty areas.

3. Besides the nursing shortage, are there other reasons why nurses have become so task-oriented?

From my observations, a number of factors have contributed to a task orientation, as shown in Table 9.1. Think about which of these concerns might apply in your organization.

Some of these factors can definitely be addressed. For instance, staff turnover is not only costly, but it contributes to being task-driven. Less experienced nurses have not yet developed expert critical thinking skills. As technology advances, we'll need more knowledge in how to operate machines and computers. The number of tasks that we do each day increases as client acuity increases. But expanding to 12-hour shifts has not guaranteed that we're more

Table 9.1 Factors That Can Contribute to Task Focus

- Focus on tasks in most basic nursing programs and for competency assessments
- Increased number of tasks to perform in less time
- Advances in technology
- Client acuity and complexity of care
- Lack of empowerment to think critically
- 12-hour shifts in inpatient settings (too many tasks to do)
- High staff turnover

productive. While seemingly convenient for the nurse's schedule, 12-hour shifts are too long and tiring. It's difficult to think when you're exhausted or haven't eaten!

Lack of empowerment is a very important issue. The age of "mama" and "papa" management, or "micro-managing," is over. The people who do the work, in this case the nurses who provide care, are in the best position to determine what clients need and how to provide their care. Managers must guide the nurses and other staff as they make their own decisions. When a staff member approaches a manager with a problem, the response should be, "What do you think you/we should do? What would you do if I weren't here?" Asking staff to bring two or three solutions for any problem they bring to management is very appropriate and empowers them to develop their critical thinking (Ignatavicius, 2001).

4. Are nurses the only healthcare professionals who have become so task-oriented?

Of course other disciplines are facing the same issues as nursing. For example, when a respiratory therapist comes on a hospital unit, he/she has a list of treatments (tasks) that have to be completed. As each one is done, it is checked off. New, inexperienced physical and occupational therapists also plan their work in a similar fashion, rather than looking at the bigger interdisciplinary picture and focusing on expected outcomes for the client. A more seasoned respiratory therapist will be discussing the impact of treatments on the plan of care, and integrating the timing with the other disciplines, such as physical therapy and nursing. Medication for pain might be a good thing to coordinate with the breathing treatment of a post-thoracotomy patient.

5. Should we expect all levels of nursing staff to think critically, including the unlicensed assistive personnel (UAP)?

We want *all* employees to think critically within their cognitive ability and scope of practice. Unlicensed nursing staff need to know and practice according to the acceptable standards of care. In other words, they should function at Level 1 (basic) in their thinking (see Chapter 5 for further discussion of levels of critical thinking). For example, we know that toileting incontinent clients every few hours helps to prevent falls. If UAP choose not to toilet the clients, they are not practicing at the basic level of thinking (see Chapter 11 for more details on UAP accountabilities).

6. I've heard some nurses complaining about lack of time to think critically. What concerns do practicing nurses have related to critical thinking?

Most nurses would agree that they are more task-oriented than outcome-oriented. Asked what they usually do to relieve clients' pain, they typically respond that they would administer pain medication. Yet, there are many options for controlling pain. It's easier to follow the healthcare provider's order for pain medication than think about what other options might be available.

Other task-oriented comments you may hear include the following:

- I'm not allowed to think; I might get in trouble. (lack of empowerment)
- They don't pay me enough to think critically. (inadequate compensation)
- I wasn't really prepared for this work. (lack of knowledge)
- Thinking takes energy, and I don't have much. (fatigue)
- I don't have time to think. (short-staffed)
- There's no incentive to think critically. (lack of reward system)
- The physicians don't want us to think; they think that's their job. (lack of understanding about nursing's role; lack of collaboration)

Obviously, if any of these concerns apply where you work, you'll want to address them. Not only do they stifle critical thinking, they can lead to high staff turnover.

7. How can we counter these concerns in our healthcare setting?

Probably the most important approach to these concerns is to create an environment that expects and appreciates critical thinking. This approach must be the philosophy throughout the organization. That means that critical thinking is expected, nurtured, fostered, and praised. The organization's leadership team needs to embrace this philosophy and ensure that it is carried out in every department, especially in the Nursing Department.

Employees who do not think critically need education about how to do so and mentoring to develop expert skills. Those who have superior critical thinking skills need to be rewarded, and not just on their performance appraisals. As professionals, nurses are attracted to work in an environment in which they are empowered to think critically and are a part of the organization's decision-making process. Empowerment, then, is a good recruitment and retention tool.

8. Speaking of recruitment and retention, do you think that the nursing shortage has contributed to the lack of critical thinking?

I feel strongly that the nursing shortage is a major factor in the lack of critical thinking. Throughout the country in every type of healthcare setting, professional nurses are being replaced with unlicensed assistive personnel (UAP). While the unlicensed staff members are usually expert in doing tasks, such as psychomotor skills, they do not have the knowledge base or experience to do high-level critical thinking. Much of the direct care is performed today by UAP, while nurses often find themselves struggling to find the time for advanced technological skills, comprehensive assessments, medication administration, and infusion therapy. I believe that the result of this time "crunch" is lack of focus on critical thinking.

9. Many nurses tell us that they have to be task-oriented because there are so many tasks that have to be done. What's wrong with doing the tasks?

As mentioned in the response to Question 1, every task has a critical thinking component. In addition, just focusing on getting the tasks done prevents nurses from being outcome-directed. Take the following example of a med-surg nurse's plan for 10:30 a.m. He has a list of "to dos" that need to be accomplished:

Rm. 408	J.R. needs pain med now
Rm. 409A	S.P. needs to have her IV restarted because she just pulled it out (again!)
Rm. 411	N.M. needs to have his dressing changed
Rm. 413B	H.W. needs his antibiotic renewed

In this example, as the nurse performs the tasks, they will be checked off and another list will be created. Yes, the nurse must perform these tasks. But, isn't it possible that some related assessments or interventions might be missed? Let's say that the woman in 409A pulled her IV out because she is acutely confused. She was admitted last night with a UTI and dehydration. *Why* does she need her IV restarted? The reason is that we are trying to ensure that she becomes rehydrated (the desired outcome). Is there anything else the nurse should do or assess related to this outcome? Of course! The nurse needs to encourage fluids and remind the UAP to push fluids as well. Assessments such as urine output and vital signs need to be performed to ensure that the patient is becoming rehydrated.

Sometimes in the haste to get the tasks done, I find that the outcome-focused thinking is missed. This is when errors can occur.

10. Some new graduates are overwhelmed and don't seem to grasp the "big picture." Why?

I think there are probably several answers to that question. One is that nursing programs may not prepare the new graduate for certain settings. For instance, all programs now include a significant amount of community-based nursing in their curricula. Only about 51% of nurses are employed by hospitals, so the rest are in the community or non-acute care setting. There's only so much clinical time in a formal nursing program. New graduates often want to work in trauma units, emergency departments, and other critical care areas. Nursing schools cannot prepare graduates for this type of nursing (nor should they). The program is accountable for producing nurse generalists, not specialists.

In addition, there is such a knowledge explosion that it is practically impossible to prepare nurses today who have much more than foundational concepts. Any attempt to cram too much content into a curriculum is disastrous because the student simply does not have time to learn it.

Another reason is that orientations/internships are typically too short and there's just too much information in them for the new graduate to absorb. I always say that new graduates have lots of "dots" of information (pieces of knowledge), but those dots are not connected. That is the role of the employer—to mentor the nurse and develop him/her to "connect the dots."

11. Nurses seem to be making more patient care errors, and disciplinary hearings in our state are increasing. Is this a result of inadequate critical thinking?

That state is not alone in finding an increase in state board disciplinary hearings. The National Council of State Boards of Nursing recently reported that hearings have increased throughout the country (personal communication, February, 2002). When the nurse is asked about why or why not the standard of care was not implemented, the answer is often, "I guess I just wasn't thinking." This response clearly tells me that critical thinking skills are not being consistently used in practice.

12. What are the most common errors that nurses make?

While we've heard a lot about medication errors in the past few years, there are other areas that get us in legal trouble. As a nursing malpractice expert witness, I find that most cases have several themes in common. The errors that I see include:

- Lack of adequate or comprehensive physical assessments (resulting in failure to detect significant changes in patient condition)
- Inadequate or inaccurate interpretation of assessment data (resulting in making false assumptions)
- Lack of adequate measures to prevent health problems or medical complications (resulting in health decline)
- Failure to implement interventions according to the standard of care (resulting in negative outcomes)

13. In general, how can we reduce errors in the Nursing Department?

I have found that the best way to reduce errors is to follow the guidelines in Table 9.2.

TABLE 9.2   Guidelines for Reducing Clinical Errors

- Hire qualified nurses who have the ability or the potential to think critically.
- Provide a thorough orientation for "seasoned" nurses.
- Provide an expanded internship program that focuses on critical thinking.
- Ensure that preceptors are experienced and competent.
- Ensure that adequate numbers of professional nurses are available for patient care.
- Plan ways to improve retention of experienced, competent nurses.
- Encourage nurses to continue learning by offering educational courses and having them attend "outside" conferences.
- Examine and improve systems within the organization that affect nursing care of patients.

14. Any ideas on how we can reduce medication errors?

Everyone seems to be working on this problem. I suggest a two-pronged approach. The first is to look at the medication administration system and supportive services. For example, what type of procedure is used by the pharmacy to ensure that the correct drug is available for the nurses to administer? Are med orders put into the computer by the physician? Or are orders hand written, allowing for transcription errors? Are medication dispensing systems used, or does the nurse have to find the drug in a med cart? Is there a system for reporting medication errors without fear of blame?

The second approach is to examine the competence and compliance of the disciplines involved in medication administration. If the dose is less than 1 mg, does the MD write 0.5 mg, for example, or just .5 mg? Does the unit secretary transcribe the order correctly? Does the nurse checking the order carefully monitor for errors? Does the nurse have a drug handbook or other resource for looking up unfamiliar drugs? Do the nurses have adequate knowledge about medications and their administration (Ignatavicius, 2000)?

Once these questions are answered and addressed where needed, med errors can be reduced. Inservice education can also help here, especially with improving drug knowledge and helping nurses feel that reporting errors won't result in disciplinary action. A good video on the subject is "Without Blame." You can get a copy by contacting Bridge Medical at (858)350-0100.

15. What are other typical negative outcomes that result from lack of critical thinking?

Unfortunately, the biggest negative outcome is malpractice cases that specify nurses as defendants. In a few cases, criminal charges have been filed, especially when a patient death results from lack of critical thinking. Nurses often become frustrated when they believe there's not time to think critically or that they aren't empowered to think critically. Then, morale declines, which ultimately negatively affects patient care and staff retention.

16. What are some resources that can help reduce nursing errors in general?

The most important resource is education. But what is really important is that we ensure that nurses actually learn and can apply the information, not just attend an inservice program or read an article. If you look at the list of common nursing errors in Question 12, you can see that education would probably have prevented them. Current articles, videos, and electronic media can assist with self-directed learning.

17. Morale seems to be declining among the nurses. Is this a common problem across the country?

In my travels I have seen an overall decline in nursing morale because of the factors discussed earlier. Most nurses believe that employers focus more on financial outcomes, while they focus more on patient care. I think we need to do a better job as a profession in helping students and nurses understand the importance of cost of care. But, I've found that we don't usually include that type of information in curricula or textbooks. In the last edition of Ignatavicius and Workman's book (2002), I added "Cost of Care" boxes to help students begin to see the value of considering healthcare costs when they are providing patient care. We need to see more of these efforts to educate nurses today.

18. Some studies have shown that poor morale results in decreased quality of care and retention. How should we address this problem?

In some places nurses are quite content and morale is good; in other organizations, angry, frustrated, and exhausted nurses are looking for work elsewhere. The key is to find out what nurses want and to eliminate as many dissatisfiers as possible. Studies on nurse retention repeatedly find that nurses want a strong say in how the unit and department are run. In other words, they want to think critically and make decisions that ultimately affect patient care. They also want to spend more time in patient care, rather than spending time doing non-nursing functions, such as transporting patients, emptying trashcans, and answering the phone. Once we ask nurses what they want and what makes them unhappy, only then can we begin to think about increasing retention and increasing morale.

The Magnet Nursing Services Recognition program of the American Nurses Credentialing Center (ANCC) designates magnet status to those healthcare organizations that demonstrate excellence in nursing practice. These organizations are better able to retain nurses because the nurses have:

- professional autonomy over their practice
- control over their practice environment, and
- effective communication with other nurses, physicians, and administrators (Jones-Schenk, 2001).

The criteria that are used by the ANCC are good ones to think about for your organization, even if the organization is not planning to apply for magnet status (see Table 9.3).

Nurses want to be recognized on a day-to-day basis for the excellent care they provide and they want to be positively rewarded as well. Oftentimes managers spend more time with problem staff rather than complimenting those nurses

TABLE 9.3 ANCC Criteria for Evaluating Nursing Practice

• Quality of nursing leadership	• Quality improvement program
• Organizational structure	• Consultation and resources
• Management style	• Community and the hospital
• Human resource policies and programs	• Nurses as teachers
• Quality of care	• Image of nursing
• Professional models of care	• Nurse-physician relationships
• Level of autonomy	• Professional career development

who are going beyond the minimum expectations. If we want to keep nurses, we must make them feel good about who they are. We must make them feel that they are equal partners on the healthcare team and within the organization.

Social events and recognitions are also important, such as Nurses Week and special continuing education opportunities with national speakers. Although costs may be an issue, grants are readily available for educational opportunities. Some organizations have special funds or foundations for these activities.

Of course, decreased morale also affects the quality of patient care, so administrations cannot ignore the importance of this assessment. The most successful healthcare organizations are those where these issues are addressed and nursing care is valued.

According to Levin (2001), nurses value these characteristics:

- Recognition
- Achievement and advancement
- Education
- Communication
- Peer relationships
- Quality of work
- Compensation

As you can see, this list is similar to the criteria for magnet status used by the ANCC. A good test might be to see if these values are recognized and nurtured in your organization. If not, then they need to be addressed to increase retention and morale.

19. What can we do about compensation for nurses?

Large recruitment bonuses are a short-term fix, not an answer for recruitment and retention. The nurses who have stayed in the organization feel slighted because they did not receive these monetary rewards. And, we know that money is now more of an incentive to nurses than ever before. So, perhaps we need to look at retention bonuses, over and beyond the merit raises. Several hospitals have started offering retention bonuses, rather than paying out large recruitment bonuses, and the nurses seem very content with this method of compensation.

Some hospitals have started externship programs in which they pay for the last portion of the student's formal education program and offer them an hourly wage in exchange for a one- to three-year commitment to work at the sponsoring hospital. I think this plan is excellent because students get a better impression of what hospital nurses do when they work 36 to 40 hours a week. It's a very "real world" experience for students.

That experience, coupled with a comprehensive internship program after they become licensed, should help ensure that the new graduates are more prepared for the work world. However, they need continual coaching and mentoring. According to Benner (1984), a nurse may need one to three years before critical thinking becomes an integral part of practice. We often expect way too much of new graduates.

RESOURCES

Alfaro-LeFevre, R. (2003). *Critical thinking in nursing: A practical approach* (3rd ed.). Philadelphia: Saunders.

Benner, P. (1984). *From novice to expert.* Menlo Park, CA: Addison-Wesley.

Ignatavicius, D. D. (2000). Asking the right questions about medication safety. *Nursing, 30*(9), 51–54.

Ignatavicius, D. D. (2001). Six critical thinking skills for at the bedside success. *Nursing Management, 32*(1), 37–39.

Ignatavicius, D. D., & Workman, M. L. (2002). *Medical-surgical nursing: A critical thinking approach to collaborative care.* Philadelphia: Saunders.

Jones-Schenk, J. (2001). How magnets attract nurses. *Nursing Management, 32*(1), 41–42.

Levin, P. M. (2001). The loyal treatment. *Nursing Management, 32*(1), 16–21.

National Council of State Boards of Nursing (**www.ncsbn.org**).

Chapter 10: Overcoming Barriers and Identifying the Resistance

"I keep the telephone of my mind open to peace, harmony, health, love and abundance. Then, whenever doubt, anxiety or fear try to call me, they keep getting a busy signal—and they'll soon forget my number."

—Edith Armstrong, storyteller

1. What are the major issues that get in the way of critical thinking?

Since critical thinking is simply a process of more in-depth and reflective thinking, it does not really seem that things would get in the way of what should be an everyday practice. However, there are times when you do not think your best, and it is helpful to be aware of those negative influences, as they will certainly affect the decisions you make, and ultimately the actions you take. I like to consider these three major types: personal, self-imposed, and environmental.

Personal barriers consist of the lack of those things that contribute to your health and well-being, as certainly the logical conclusion would be that it takes a healthy frame of mind and body to achieve the optimum in thought processes. Think of the times you do not feel your best, and are tired, hungry, stressed, and perhaps not in the best emotional state either. Similar to Maslow's hierarchy, you must have those basic needs satisfied in order to reach the state of self-actualization, the pinnacle of critical thinking.

You may choose not to risk your current comfort level by rocking the boat, and therefore may impose your own limits, or barriers. Recalling a past experience when you spoke up, offering creative suggestions outside of the box, and were "shot down" may cause you to withhold the results of your critical thinking analysis of future problems. A desire to be like others, and to "go with the flow" may supersede your need to be heard, and another wall will go up as you protect your group membership.

Environmental issues are a bit trickier, and may have a good deal to do with the organizational climate and culture where you are working, or the environment of family, friends, and community. Certainly there can be cultural barriers in terms of the lack of opportunity to speak out (if you are the low person in the hierarchy and there are formal limits to your being heard). Likewise, if creative thinking and openness to alternatives, as well as reflection and thinking out loud are not encouraged, but are discouraged in a "do as you are told" environment, there will be distinct barriers to critical thinking.

2. We had some consultants work with unit staff and they provided a step-by-step model for both leadership and staff to use in problem solving. The idea was for everyone to use a similar method, and increase the awareness of thinking critically. So far, no one has used it—how come?

Similar to the discussion above, the barriers may come from many directions. I like to use the checklist in Table 10.1 to discuss how the organization is doing in carrying out some of the more specific strategies for supporting critical thinking. If these things are not done, it does not matter how many models are developed by consultants. Critical thinking cannot be mandated, and a model is not a panacea for leadership that does not actively participate and demonstrate

Table 10.1: How Does Your Organization Measure Up?

- The organization believes that progress is made through the open sharing of **questions, new ideas, and risk-taking from all levels.**
- Critical thinking is **modeled by managers**, and emphasis is placed on a coaching approach with demonstrations of critical thinking behaviors in all leadership and staff meetings.
- Administrative leadership **values the need to continuously develop employees**, and demonstrates this by supporting education through tuition grants, offering education, and funding attendance at national conferences and workshops.
- **Education** works with leadership and staff to **maximize learning opportunities** through case studies and analysis of existing problems and errors.
- It is "socially acceptable" **to think through situations and problems with the assistance of a manager or peer** (i.e., it is okay to ask for help, both on a physical and cognitive level).
- **Education evaluates its effectiveness** through demonstrated learning and measurement of application impact, not focusing on the numbers of attendees in a program.
- There is a **structured mentor/preceptor program** that includes training in the processes of asking questions and encouraging thinking out loud.
- **Multidisciplinary teams** share their experiences and work together with open communication so that learning can take place across disciplines.

Note. From "Sharpening Your Critical Thinking Skills," by S. P. Kyzer, 1996, *Orthopaedic Nursing, 15*(6), p. 71. Copyright 1996 by the National Association of Orthopaedic Nurses. Adapted with permission.

critical thinking behaviors. Remember, critical thinking is a continual way of approaching issues, not an additional approach that is dusted off and used once in a while for the tough problems.

3. I am a relatively new manager, and I have read about critical thinking attitudes. They sound great on paper, but I am having difficulty seeing how to actually apply them. Do you have any specific suggestions?

What sounds great on paper, when describing concepts, often is not translated to a way that can be applied in a work setting. What does a list of attitudes mean to the manager reading all about them? Should managers hire people like this, or can these attitudes be developed in existing staff? I have created a list of applications that I share with managers as we discuss very specific approaches they may take to make the concept "real."

- **Intellectual integrity** (true to your own thoughts and consistent in standards):

  Are you consistent in your treatment of others? Does the staff see you as impartial, or practicing a degree of favoritism? Do you have a separate set of rules for your own conduct or is it the same for both management and staff?

- **Intellectual humility and suspending judgment** (sensitive to bias, prejudice, and limitation of views, okay to say "I don't know," and to recognize the foundation of one's beliefs):

  Are you willing to "suspend judgment" and to be approachable in terms of a situation that you may not have first hand experience with? Can you, and do you, role model by clarifying to others the basis of your belief or opinion?

- **Fair-minded and open to other points of view** (reconstruct accurately the views of others and to reason from ideas other than our own):

  When dealing with interpersonal conflict, do you ask the individual to state the other's position, and then seek clarification from that individual (what is Ted angry about? Ted, is that right?)?

- **Make interdisciplinary connections** (recognize the arbitrary distinctions between disciplines, whether they are academic [nursing vs. English vs. the arts] or departmental [nursing vs. pharmacy vs. radiology]):

  Take every opportunity to include the views of all of the other departments by having representatives attend staff meetings, or shift reports. Encourage discussion of outside interests, today's news, and examples in other industries that may have similar implications for nursing.

- **Support the power of questioning** (see questions as an opportunity to develop a line of thought and to help learn what others are thinking):

Support the development of thought by asking questions, not just making statements and dispensing news. When having a staff meeting, or case discussion, be sure to summarize using a Socratic technique: "We began with this question, and some of you said _____, others said _____. Let's look at the pros and cons of both issues and continue. Our goal is to establish a consensus about this topic."

4. It's pretty hard to sustain an inquiring attitude when it seems that questioning just rocks the boat. Who wants the extra stress of being labeled as a troublemaker?

No question that questioning rocks the boat. An important ingredient of an environment that supports critical thinking is rewards for critical thinking—rewards and support for "boat rocking." And perseverance in questioning can actually begin to make that change—if leaders truly commit to building an environment that fosters critical thinking. For example, reward the reporting of errors rather than only rewarding error-free practice; show openness to alternative ways of doing things—new assignments for UAP, alternative working hours, job-sharing, and the like.

Make questioning a habit. Like any other habit, repeated practice is necessary to cement the habit in place. Once you have incorporated the attitude of inquiry into your approach, there will be no stopping the questions. And many of them will stimulate positive changes.

Reflect on the success of your questioning technique. Do you need to take a different tack? For example, rather than advocating a change in practice by saying, "I think the way we did those dressings where I used to work was much better," try, "You really do a great job with those dressings here. Another good technique we used where I used to work was . . . The advantage was . . . What do you think of that approach?" When you reflect on the success of your questioning technique, you are actually using critical thinking to enhance your critical thinking approach. Or as critical thinking authorities Paul and Heaslip (1995) suggested thinking about your thinking while you are thinking to make your thinking better: more clear, more accurate, or more defensible.

When you raise a question, try to offer at least one answer or suggestion along with the question. In a way, questions identify problems or potential problems. The receiver of this kind of communication usually welcomes the question more receptively if you propose a constructive suggestion.

While you are persisting in your questioning and waiting for the environment to truly embrace critical thinking, build your own critical thinking support system.

Identify, interact with, and cultivate relationships with people who share your value of the attitude of inquiry. For further suggestions to sustain critical thinking in the face of skeptics, see Brookfield's (1993) article.

5. How can I respond when nurses tell me that critical thinking is a luxury—a nice-to-know versus a need-to-know?

Show them the value of critical thinking applied to the issues *they identify*. If they perceive that they barely have time to get the essential care accomplished, that's the place to start. What distractions or tasks that they might delegate are eroding their control over their time? What activities are consuming most of their time? Help them analyze the contributors to the lack of time.

Avoid rushing to solutions. Be sure that you've identified all aspects of the problem before you devise a solution. Consider discrete changes that attack specific aspects of the problem. For example: What geographical, logistic or systems changes could alleviate their frustration? What other assignment strategies could help?

6. The charge nurse says we are too busy to take time and sit and discuss patient treatment and care plans. I'm frustrated, and I wonder what can be done.

This reminds me of that old saying, "If you fail to plan, then plan to fail." Likewise, if you do not have time to discuss patient treatment and plans among the care team, what do you have time for? There are so many reasons that we fall into the task mentality, seek to complete the visible and measurable work, and forego the thinking component. Much of the essential work of the staff occurs on the fly, as staff grab a moment here and there to share an idea, run something by a colleague, and seek validation for what they are planning to do.

What assumptions are you making about the charge nurse and her priorities, based on her statement that you are too busy to discuss plans? Perhaps it is time to seek some clarification about what she is thinking. What does the charge nurse see as most important? How would she like to see care planned and discussed? Is the unit manager in agreement? What are you doing now to share ideas and plans about patient care?

Time is one of the most significant barriers/excuses/rationales for the choices we make and the actions we are or are not taking. Priorities guide decisions only if we are clear about what the fundamental values are, the desired outcomes, and how our actions will achieve those outcomes. I think the best way to make time for this kind of sharing is to discuss the situation with the charge nurse, and the rest of the staff, and determine what you are spending time on, and what is most important.

7. I know critique is an important part of critical thinking. Most nurses don't want to engage in constructive critique. They're afraid of the consequences of criticizing the nurses they work with, but they're ready to criticize the staff on other shifts. How can I increase their willingness to engage in constructive criticism?

Unfortunately, the nursing culture is such that "criticism" will never be welcomed—at least not in the foreseeable future. We have too much history of punitive discipline to suddenly embrace criticism of our own individual practice and performance. But, critique is an important part of critical thinking and an important part of improving practice and patient care.

Call upon the critical thinking skill of reframing. It sounds like the terms critique and criticism create too much resistance. Remove the threat that criticism of individual performance implies. Focus on the indicators of outcomes you are attempting to monitor and improve, such as labeling IV tubing, or documenting patients' response to pain medication.

First orient the nurses to the focus (focus on indicators of care, not on individual performance). Then, use objective monitoring tools to collect data and report the results back to the staff. Let them raise suggestions about how to improve and how to facilitate compliance. Implement some of their suggestions. With this preparation, the nurses may be ready to collect data using the monitoring tools. At this point, the focus is clearly on improvement of care and practice.

Nurses form impressions of one another's practice as they work together. Some of these impressions may be based on false assumptions or biases. Constructive critique or criticism is based upon specific, clear, objective criteria. Keep the focus on the criteria and how those criteria support safe, effective care and professional practice.

Some facilities have successfully incorporated peer review programs into their professional development systems. Success rests, at least in part, on clear criteria and orientation to peer review by taking preparatory steps similar to those described in Chapter 13 regarding stress relief.

8. My manager asks me to "think out loud" and to explain why I did what I did in terms of treating the patient, or working with the staff. I hate to do that, and am afraid she is going to find out that I don't really know what I am doing. How can I get around this?

I would bet that this situation reminds you of being in math class when the teacher said to "show your work"! That is really what this is all about; trying to find ways to make thinking visible so that we can all continue to learn where our judgments come from, and what assumptions and data are being used to come to the decisions that we ultimately act upon. I think it is a very important first step that you have recognized that your fear is "being found out," and that you may be shattering that illusion that you think others have of you being the clinical expert. In actuality, thinking out loud is a highly expert practice, as it allows others to see how you are processing information. If you consider that point of view, it may help you understand that by taking a risk, you are really modeling an important critical behavior and assisting others to grow by comparison and mentoring. Yes, this is risk taking, and you may want to minimize the risk by prefacing your comments with that disclaimer, "I am not sure this is right, and this is how I look at what information there is…" If the manager is supportive and thinking critically as well, she will realize that there is no "right" process, and encourage you to continue. If she is not supportive, it is time for you to share your reluctance, discuss your concerns about not being thought correct, and identify specifically what you need in order to become more comfortable in thinking out loud.

9. Do you have suggestions on how to implement changes that we learn about outside of work?

One of the fundamental barriers to change is lack of personal connection and motivation. You may attend a conference, be relaxed and in a comfortable environment, and find yourself excited and energized by the ideas that are shared. Remember, that while you were gone, the staff continued to work in the same conditions, with the same stressors, and did not have the opportunity for renewal and excitement that you did. In order to have some success at sharing and implementing any new ideas that you learned, you will need to appeal to the motivation of your colleagues.

Consider frames of reference, and the differences between what you heard at the workshop and how it would be perceived and applied in your work setting.

Each member of the team is going to be considering your information through the personal filter, WIIFM, What's In It For Me? Have you thought specifically about how the proposed change will benefit others, and what it will mean in terms of what they have to do differently? Often change will involve giving up something that was familiar, and therefore easier. The new approach and concept will certainly require adjustment and additional work until it becomes a practiced process. It will be essential to be clear regarding the benefits while acknowledging the work of the change itself.

10. **In report, we often hear the opinions of the staff who have taken care of the patients on the previous shift, and this may affect the way we interact with the patients. I do not really want to know that "Mrs. Jones is noncompliant," or that "Mr. Smith is just one of those demanding attorneys that you have to watch out for," or that "Mrs. White is just trying to get more drugs—she really doesn't have any pain." How do I tune out these comments?**

Report is the time for sharing information that will assist the next team in continuing the care of the patients in a consistent manner. Unfortunately, being social animals, the gathering of the troops also results in a time when personal opinions are shared and often serve to validate the work of the caregivers (look at me, this was a tough shift, and this patient is a real challenge!). As we learned in psych classes, this kind of indirect request for feedback and recognition is important to sustain the positive team behaviors we want, but if it comes at the expense of the patient, it will be more detrimental than intended.

I think the more effective approach is not to tune out opinionated comments, and instead, to understand why they are being shared, and what you can do to either change that or to respond in such a way that directs the report to more factual information. Remember, it is only your behavior that you can control, and not the other individual's. The best you can hope for from the colleague who shares personal judgments regarding patient behaviors and motives, is to bring this to his attention, and be specific about how this may set you up (the classic self-fulfilling policy), and prejudice you to look for behaviors in the patient that may not really be true when you care for the patient.

You might suggest that report be changed to one that is in front of the patient, including the patient in the dialogue, and seeking clarification from patient and family if the care that is planned is in agreement with their desired outcomes.

You may also suggest that if report is taped that a format be developed to structure the information that is shared, so that more factual exchanges occur.

11. **The last new hire that we oriented had some great suggestions for doing things differently. Her ideas were shot down immediately with an emphatic "that's not the way we do things here!" She did not stay very long. How do we help people to see that there are new ways that can work better?**

It sounds like your culture wants to preserve the status quo, even when reminded that the status may long have diminished and would benefit from a different approach. It sounds like you have some work to do in terms of data gathering and interpretation. Was this resistance limited to this new orientee only, or is there a pattern of treating all new orientees in a similar manner? Once you have determined if this is an isolated response, or a more general attitude that the department has, you will have a better idea of how to proceed. I would suggest one of the models discussed in Chapter 4 would help you with the steps of problem solving with the rest of the staff.

12. **When I ask one of the staff to explain what or why, or the reason behind his/her action, I am met with a defensive response, and usually the person shrugs me off. What can I do to get him/her thinking?**

It may depend on how you are asking the question. Perhaps the place to start is a careful review of your approach, as that is the only thing you can control. Be sure you have a neutral tone in your voice, and are not implying in any way that you believe that this person is wrong. Remember that a critical thinking approach is to keep an open mind and to appreciate the differences in perspectives that others will have. Reflect on a situation in which you asked a staff member to explain his thinking. Recall exactly what you said, where you were, and what your purpose was in asking the question in the first place. If the nurse was in the middle of considering two patient requests, and anticipating the transfer of a third, your timing may have been off. At a busy work setting, with numerous other colleagues around, she may have felt on the spot, regardless of the tone of your voice. While your intent may have been to model critical inquiry, and encourage thinking out loud, the best place to start will be in a quiet and individual space. This is especially true if you know, or have reason to suspect, a defensive response.

Again, turn the situation around and remember how you feel when the supervisor asks you to explain your actions. How does it feel? If you find yourself comfortable and not feeling defensive, reflect on what style the supervisor is using to allow you to have this comfort level. If you find that you are feeling just as defensive as the staff member you are concerned about, it is time to sit down and discuss your rationale for asking these questions, what the purpose is, and how you can make it more comfortable for both of you.

13. One of the members of the team is always exaggerating. Any suggestions for how to make her a little more intellectually honest?

I think it is important to understand what is driving this behavior in the first place. Consider this example: "I really do not like working with Mary. She *never* offers to take a new patient, she is *always* complaining and *seldom* does she really do anything to help out. *Every* time I have discussed this with the manager, she tells me she will talk to Mary, but so far, *nothing* has changed." This is a classic example! I have discovered that the vague and exaggerated generalities of the person who is frustrated by another's performance are symptoms of a need to make the case seem important in order to prompt corrective action, and to make sure that I see that it is such a problem that I will be eager to take care of it immediately.

What do you think might be reasons that your colleague is exaggerating? A careful consideration of your own assumptions, attitudes, and why this situation exists will be time well spent in clarifying the issue and helping you determine what is the best action to take. What questions can you ask this person that will help her be more specific? I would suggest acknowledging what she is saying ("Yes, I know that this kind of patient can be very difficult." "I realize working with someone who does not offer help when you need it can be frustrating."). Then ask her for a specific example of what she is describing. ("Can you give me a specific example of what you are talking about? That would really help me to determine what I should be doing.")

Some people grow up in a culture of exaggeration and of telling colorful stories. Part of it may be a means of gaining attention and being heard, and the exaggerations may be just a cultural expectation that is part of this individual's personality. You may not change the exaggerator, but you can help to get beyond the embellishments and to the specifics you need in order to respond and take action. Begin by being the clarifier, identifying clearly what you need.

14. **How do you deal with emotions? Sometimes the staff is so angry and upset, particularly during busy times or at a staff meeting, and we do not get anywhere. And one nurse always dissolves into tears whenever anyone challenges her.**

> Tears and anger are two emotions that find their way into the healthcare setting frequently. In the intense environment of caring for people, there is plenty of opportunity for the feeling side to be more visible than in other work environments. Feelings are a fundamental part of who we are, as in these two quotes: "I felt before I thought" (Rousseau), and "Feeling is first" (e.e. cummings). However, the message from society is to leave emotion out of it. I have certainly heard more than one administrative leader say to park your emotions at the door. Impossible to do, and certainly not part of critical thinking! Critical thinkers will understand that emotions are part of all that we do, and do not represent personal barriers, although they may be hurdles to get over on the way to clarified problem solving. I suggest using the work of Goleman (2000) regarding emotional intelligence, and discussing emotional control with those who are having difficulties. Sometimes an open conversation about the tears, and the anger, helps to find out what is underneath the emotion, after the storm has passed.
>
> Remember, once again, those critical thinking concepts of validating your assumptions, and being clear about your frame of reference. Some people are very uncomfortable around emotional expressions, and others appear to just ignore it and move on. I am not sure that either approach is ideal, although I would suggest that you be clear regarding the effect on you, and what you need to do to be able to neutralize the situation. One good thing about emotional displays is the idea that you are clear about what the person is feeling! Then the challenge becomes finding out *why*.

15. **There usually seems to be one person on the team who is negative about everything, no matter what. Are there any strategies for dealing with this person so the rest of us can try some creative problem solving?**

> Similar to the person who shoots holes in all of your ideas, this individual can be helping to identify the weak components in your plan. However, if the predominant attitude is a generalized negative approach, then it is time to sit down with that person and discuss what his goals are in relationship to the work unit. Finding out what is important to him will assist you both in determining what

changes can be made to improve your communication efforts. A specific example describing a time when he is negative will help you to illustrate what you are concerned about, and provide something to respond to in terms of behavior and rationale.

Remember that the term "negative about everything" is your perception, and may not be his. He may actually think that he is not being critical, and is even being helpful in pointing out the things that are not working.

16. Documentation is always a big issue for us, but despite continued efforts, there are those staff who don't seem to think before they write. What can I do?

Documentation is indeed a big issue, and there are just as many reasons and differences in the process as there are in shift report. Why do we document? Ideally, the medical record is created to be a permanent form of communication among all disciplines, usually regarding the care of patients. However, it is so much more than that. Staff will acknowledge the famous teaching, "if it isn't charted, it wasn't done," making documentation an opportunity to provide proof of all of the work we have done on the patient's behalf. It is also a means for self-protection, as the prevailing opinion is one of "CYA," to use the current phrase. These two themes have created a process in which the nurse will use a checklist mentality to include observations and actions performed on the patient's behalf, and will seldom include that next step of demonstrating the judgment and critical thinking that take place in order to validate the plan of care. The classic laundry list of patient assessment data is important as a baseline, but the key component becomes what is done with that data.

In response to your question, it is possible to teach staff to think before they write and to make changes in the direction and intent of the documentation itself. It will only occur as a unified and systematic effort, however, and not through the individual work of one leader who would like to see improvements. The following steps may help to develop critical charting:

- Review the current processes and the policies that support them.
- Review records through the use of an audit tool (Joint Commission on Accreditation of Healthcare Organizations [JCAHO] has a fairly comprehensive one, and you may also want to tailor one to your specific concerns).
- Have a team of nurses use the tool to review charts and see for themselves what is being documented.

- Review nurses notes individually; have management take an active role in daily review.

- Develop and use examples of what are desired notations that reflect thinking in action and include the analysis of patient responses to treatment, linked to continuous plans of care.

- Read the article, "Charting Critical Thinking: Nursing Judgments and Patient Outcomes," by Chase (1997).

17. I have used the "Socratic Dialogue" process in staff meetings and with task forces. Sometimes it works, but sometimes someone just shrugs, gets embarrassed, and does not want to respond. The rest of the team is embarrassed too, and then the discussion deteriorates. Any ideas?

The Socratic Dialogue can be a handy method to use to ensure that everyone has an opportunity to participate in the discussion, while creating an expectation of attentive listening. I use an adaptation of the method described by Richard Paul (**www.criticalthinking.org**). Briefly, the process includes these steps: let everyone know that you are practicing Socratic responsiveness, and that as facilitator, you will be guiding the discussion. Let them also know that the expectation will be to build on the previous person's statements, because before you can add your input, you will need to paraphrase what has been said so far, checking with the previous speaker to see if you have it right. There is a heightened awareness of what is being said, because as the facilitator, you may call on anyone to speak next and so no one knows when his/her "turn" will come. After doing this for about 5–10 minutes, debrief by asking how everyone felt, what was different about this style of discussion, and was their listening more effective. You will find it takes a good deal of energy—but is a great exercise!

Staff have told me that this process can be very intimidating, particularly to those who are not comfortable speaking up, and to those groups that are not normally supportive of each other. The key to this would be to begin slowly, be very clear about the "rules," and do a short demonstration with volunteers who have agreed to participate. You might also ask some of the folks who are typically the quiet ones to prepare a couple of comments prior to the meeting. The goal of this process is to discuss many sides of an issue, allowing all to share and know that they will be listened to, and certainly not to make anyone feel uncomfortable. As you have noted, once that happens, the conversation will deteriorate and the focus will shift to the emotions of the person who is struggling. You might state at the beginning that if anyone you call on does not want to speak, he/she may reserve the right to remain silent. However, you will then want to work with this person privately, coaching him/her to make sure that his/her voice and opinions are valued and heard.

18. When someone raises an issue that could be worked on in our department, several of the staff will have a defeatist attitude and claim that nothing ever changes, so why bother anyway? How can I get them past this defeatist barrier?

No doubt, that is a tough one! Defeatist attitudes can paralyze thinking and more importantly drag down morale until there is virtually no growth, and then truly nothing ever changes. One thing that I find helpful is to lead an exercise in identifying problems in terms of solvability. So often, nurses will define problems in ways they have no control or influence over, and therefore perpetuate the feeling of helplessness.

For example, if the community is in the midst of a snowstorm, and all roads are blocked, making it impossible for more staff to come in and assist at the health-care facility, defining the problem as "we need more staff" is a setup for failure. Likewise, if you are starting a new shift, with two fewer people than staffing guidelines suggest, and the supervisor tells you that everyone has been called, and there are no available staff, how would you define the problem? If you state that the problem is "not enough staff," the solution can only be to get more staff, and you have already been told that all resources have been exhausted. How else could you define the situation? Consider what effects the staffing limitations have on the ability to deliver care. Evaluate your assumptions and frame of reference as well. If you consider that you "are short two people," the inherent assumption is that the staffing guideline is a fundamental law, and that you are working in a deficit situation. Are you really? How do you know that the care required of the current patient population equals what two more staff would provide? What information do you need at this point to better define the problem?

In the situation above, it may be that a careful review of the status of the patients indicates that the staff available will be able to meet the needs of the patients, if you readjust some priorities, and assign the staff into teams. The problem may really have become, how do we reassign work based on patient priorities so that we can meet the needs of the patients and feel good about our work?

One of the aspects of critical thinking is being aware of the frame of reference you are using and the impact it has on the interpretation of the data available. Once again, questions help clarify the existing situation and reduce the negativity of a "what's the use?" attitude.

19. **One of the more senior members of the staff, both in terms of age and experience, is very hard to work with when it comes to discussing new ideas. She always thinks she is right (often she is) and therefore, she shoots holes in every new idea. What can we do, short of leaving her out of the discussions entirely?**

This can be a very frustrating situation for both sides of the discussion! I like to use a general exercise that helps to build better relationships before you disintegrate into a conflict over adapting a new idea. Consider sitting down with this person and sharing some personal information, such as family news, what you like to do when you are not working, or what books you read. Once she has shared in kind, move onto talking about ways you both sometimes feel misunderstood, either by a colleague at work, or a friend, or a family member. Then talk specifically about how each of you misunderstands the other in terms of trying a new idea. Write down what you hear her saying, and have her write down what she hears you saying. Review each other's descriptions and clarify or correct if you are not in agreement with what has been written. You may be surprised at the key issues that are uncovered and the reasons why she appears to be so resistant to new ideas.

There are several good things about having this kind of individual on the team: she plays the devil's advocate, and helps to identify areas where the proposed change may have difficulties; she is willing to share experience and voice her opinion, rather than resorting to silent sabotage; and as you note, she is often right!

20. **Staff nurses are getting older, and the workforce is aging in general. How do we continue to renew and adapt to the changing work environment and keep the more senior staff engaged?**

This is an issue that faces us in all areas, and not just the healthcare work setting. In the midst of the aging baby boomer population, it seems that everywhere you turn are people over 50 who have been in their respective work roles for over 20 years. While this seasoned experience can be a good thing, it can also mean that there is a higher element of resistance to change, and a danger in perpetuating traditions that are no longer appropriate or effective. Turn this around for a minute, and consider the opposite perspective. It may also mean that after doing things one way for so long, the senior nurse may be a bit bored and ready for some new approaches!

I find it helpful to consider a specific practice, such as patient teaching, and engage the more seasoned nurses in a review of what they have done in their past experiences to assist patients in better understanding their condition and treatment. I will then partner the senior member with a younger staff who is active on the Internet, and have the younger staff member share some of the latest interactive sites and tools available for patient reference, as well as some of the things recently discussed in school.

RESOURCES

Brookfield, S. (1993). On impostership, cultural suicide and other dangers: How nurses learn about critical thinking. *The Journal of Continuing Education in Nursing, 24*(5), 197–205.

Chase, S. K. (1997). Charting critical thinking: Nursing judgments and patient outcomes. *Dimensions of Critical Care Nursing, 16*(2), 102–111.

Goleman, D. (2000*). Working with emotional intelligence*. New York: Bantam Books.

Kyzer, S. P. (1996). Sharpening your critical thinking skills. *Orthopaedic Nursing, 15*(6), 66–76.

Paul, R. W., & Heaslip, P. (1995). Critical thinking and intuitive nursing practice. *Journal of Advanced Nursing, 22*, 40–47.

Section 3:
Putting the Elephant to Work: Practical Applications in the Field of Health Care

Employing critical thinking methods in practice has one huge barrier: nurses themselves. Once in practice we often feel a sense of arrival and, thus, stability and acceptance. Therefore, challenges are met with resistance. This section offers many useful approaches for staff, managers, educators, and clinical nurse specialists to consider in nudging educators and other healthcare colleagues along. Since critical thinking is an evolving process, it is reasonable to expect all of us to learn new ways to make better clinical judgments.

11. Individual and Organizational Accountabilities
Bette Case, PhD, RN, BC

12. Setting Priorities
Bette Case, PhD, RN, BC

13. Selecting Practice Issues for Critical Thinking Application
Bette Case, PhD, RN, BC

14. Collaborating for Effective Resolution
Bette Case, PhD, RN, BC

15. Evidence-Based Practice
Bette Case, PhD, RN, BC

16. Research and the Role of Critical Thinking and Clinical Judgment
Elizabeth E. Hand, MS, RN, CCRN

Chapter 11: Individual and Organizational Accountabilities

"Progress is impossible without change, and those who cannot change their minds cannot change anything."

—George Bernard Shaw, 1856–1950, British playwright and novelist

1. What does it mean to be accountable for clinical judgment and critical thinking?

It's helpful to think of accountability for clinical judgment and critical thinking in the same way that we think about accountability for the customer service aspect of our practice and the organization's business. Organizations that deliver outstanding customer service (in healthcare or in any other industry) take the position that customer service is everybody's business. And so it is with critical thinking.

It's important to define the roles and responsibilities of each level of staff with respect to clinical judgment and critical thinking. But no one should be excluded from the expectation of critical thinking within the scope of his/her job.

Each member of the organization, and that includes executive and board members, is accountable for using best judgment within the scope of his/her job description. For staff in entry level positions (in both clinical and non-clinical departments), critical thinking and judgment are limited to:

- making decisions about basic safety issues
- recognizing that something is wrong
- recognizing if and when an exception can be made
- identifying the need to report a situation to a supervisor
- applying some basic communication techniques in interactions with patients, family, and staff members
- understanding a problem from the point of view of another, a patient's family member for example, and taking that concern to the proper person

That last point reminds me of a recent newspaper account of an elderly woman in Wisconsin who was trapped by an automatic newspaper machine outside a drugstore. She was wearing a winter jacket and the tie of her hood got caught in the door of the newspaper vending machine after she removed a newspaper. She was trapped in an awkward position and lacked the physical flexibility to remove her jacket. She was relieved when a store employee approached. But when she asked the person to insert a couple of quarters in the coin slot to open the door and free her, the employee insisted on holding the line on "No refunds." The woman endured a long, cold, frustrating ordeal before the employee finally relented. Fortunately, the store management and the newspaper apologized and made modest reparations.

That story illustrates that even, and maybe especially, employees who have little formal training and work in entry level positions need to be expected to think—to see the situation from the viewpoint of the other party and to consider "Is this a situation in which an exception is needed? I'll ask my supervisor." Notice that I'm not recommending that any staff member overstep the boundaries of his/her competency by taking any action other than to report the situation and ask for help.

One of the safety issues that arises frequently with unlicensed assistive personnel (UAP) is when to ask for help—to report something unexpected or to ask for physical assistance in getting a heavy patient out of bed.

Each member of the staff is accountable for his/her own thinking and judgment and answerable for the results. Holding staff members answerable for the results of their thinking and judgment is a management role—enforcing the expectation of judgment and thinking with rewards and consequences.

The organizational leadership is accountable for:

- setting expectations
- supporting managers in holding staff accountable for expectations
- role modeling critical thinking and sound judgment
- establishing an atmosphere in which inquiry, curiosity, and challenge are welcomed and rewarded

Ideally, the organizational leadership adopts, or adapts, and communicates a model of critical thinking and, with the input of managers, translates the model into specific behaviors appropriate to each department and each level. But even in the absence of an endorsed model, critical thinking behaviors and attitudes can be translated into job expectations.

2. I understand that it should be a top-down initiative in an organization, but the executives here have other priorities. How can I get them interested?

Learn all that you can about those other priorities. Show the boss how critical thinking strategies address the priorities. For example, if nurse staffing is a priority, employ some of the strategies suggested in the recruitment and retention section of this book. Or, suggest some strategies for reframing short-staffing situations and getting needed assistance.

Take every opportunity to point out how staff can improve care, reduce errors, and diminish other safety risks by using specific critical thinking strategies. Preaching the value of critical thinking will not help. Instead, demonstrate the positive results of critical thinking skills.

3. Can I realistically expect organizational leadership to get involved in promoting and supporting critical thinking?

Yes—when you demonstrate results of critical thinking that are important to leadership. Then recommend more improvements available through enhanced critical thinking skills. For example, many organizations are focusing on forging more solid relationships with their communities. Critical thinking strategies such as clarifying multiple perspectives and collaborating can facilitate stronger relationships with the community. And those same strategies can prove effective in internal initiatives involving interdisciplinary collaboration and quality/performance improvement.

4. What is a Chief Nurse Executive's role in accountability for clinical judgment and critical thinking?

A Chief Nurse Executive sets the climate. The nursing leader:

- fosters the attitude of inquiry
- encourages staff to challenge assumptions
- role models critical thinking strategies and skills—and thinks out loud while doing so to make the process explicit for others
- expects those whom he/she supervises to think critically and enforces that expectation with rewards and consequences
- models and expects effective collaboration

5. What kinds of nurse manager behaviors support a critical thinking environment?

- Identify the specific outcomes and evidences of critical thinking and clinical judgment that contribute to safe, high quality care on the unit.
- When you interview applicants, pose situations for them that often occur on the unit and require critical thinking behaviors. Ask applicants how they would handle those situations. They won't know the unit policies, but that's not the point of asking the question. You are assessing their thought process.

- When you appraise performance, offer praise for evidence of those essential critical thinking behaviors—and give constructive critical feedback when you observe absence of those behaviors. Don't wait for formal performance appraisal. Commit to giving feedback specific to critical thinking behaviors on a daily basis.

- When you introduce new policies and procedures, ask staff what problems they had with the old way of doing things. Connect their complaints to improvements in the new policy. Compare and contrast the new way with the old way rather than simply presenting the new way.

- When staff members bring you problems, challenge them to identify their criteria for an acceptable solution. Challenge them to examine the way in which they have defined the problem—are there other possible ways to define it? For example, is the problem really that too many patients have been assigned to the nurse? Or might it be that the nurse does not trust the UAP to perform tasks that could lighten the nurse's work load? This will help prevent the frustration of solving the wrong problem.

- When conducting meetings, always challenge yourself to identify why a meeting is the best way to achieve the desired outcome. Meetings are a very expensive method of getting things done and the cost/benefit ratio is often unfavorable. If a meeting is indeed necessary—who needs to be there? How long does the meeting need to last? How much time will you allot to each specific outcome? How will you follow up on implementation of the decisions reached at the meeting?

- When you make rounds, take along a critical thinking question and ask it of every staff member you encounter. "What goal is most important to this patient today?" "What parameters are you monitoring most closely with this patient today?" "What is your goal for this patient today?" "How is this patient different from other patients we usually see on the unit?"

- Participate actively in interdisciplinary efforts by clarifying and examining the assumptions you make from the nursing perspective and encouraging other parties to do the same.

- Develop the habit of asking rather than telling. When you give corrective feedback to staff, ask the staff member to identify what's wrong with the approach he/she is taking. For example, "What's the risk in the way you're doing that?" "What might happen if you continue to . . .?"

- Encourage staff to identify and raise ethical questions related to patient care.

- Role model an openness to alternatives and a healthy skepticism that there is only one right way of doing things.

- Most important, encourage an ongoing environment of curiosity. Visualize a big inflated question mark floating around the unit and hovering over puzzling situations—or situations in which there are opportunities for improvement. Challenge yourself to keep that question mark aloft.

6. Does the Joint Commission on Accreditation of Healthcare Organizations (JCAHO) hold us accountable for critical thinking?

You won't find Standards like CT1.1.1 if that's what you mean. However, many JCAHO requirements connect with critical thinking. The competencies that JCAHO requires you to identify, validate, and document should include those related to critical thinking and clinical judgment. Another example is the process of root cause analysis which JCAHO requires in response to sentinel events. Organizational performance improvement requirements also require the kind of inquiry, analysis, and generation of alternatives that is at the heart of critical thinking.

7. For what is the nurse accountable?

Every nurse is accountable for safe, effective, legal, and ethical practice. But it is up to the clinical manager to translate those broad accountabilities into specific actions that relate to the scope of care on any given clinical unit. The manager is responsible for clarifying these expectations—beginning in orientation, continuing with ongoing feedback, both corrective and positive, and periodically summarizing progress in performance appraisal. The manager is also responsible for ensuring that these accountabilities include the specific elements of clinical judgment and critical thinking that are most important to patient care on the unit.

8. How can I keep my own critical thinking skills sharp?

- Reflect on the situations in which you've been involved and taken action. Critical thinking authority Richard Paul (1995) defined critical thinking as thinking about your thinking while you are thinking in order to make your thinking better: more clear, more accurate, or more defensible. Engage in reflective review and critique of your actions.

- Make an inquiring attitude part of your approach. Ask questions such as "What's wrong with this picture?" "What am I assuming here?" "Are those assumptions valid in this situation?" "What else do I need to know?" "What else can we try?"

- Offer to and seek support from others who are challenging themselves to grow in their critical thinking proficiency. Reflect on situations together. Examine issues from as many perspectives as you can describe.

- Look for alternatives. Not only "What else might we do?" but also "Who else needs to be involved?" "Where else can we look for answers?"
- Pride yourself in identifying evidence to support your conclusions—or even better, to justify a change in your viewpoint.

9. As a nurse manager I keep hearing from the director that she sees too many unusual occurrence/incident reports that show staff nurses just aren't thinking. I discipline them but what else can I do?

You're asking an important critical thinking question when you ask, "What else?" You're demonstrating the attitude of inquiry if you're sincere in wanting to explore some alternatives. Critical thinking strategies offer some important ways to treat mistakes and prevent them in the future.

Make an example of the mistake and not the nurse who made it. Let the mistake be an occasion to get staff involved in an informal root cause analysis. Use a staff meeting to probe with successive "Why?" questions. Persist until you get to the root of the problem. If a medication error occurs and you ask why it happened, you may learn that the nurse was distracted.

But that's only the beginning—why was the nurse distracted? Continue until you have reached the most basic causes of the problem. Then begin identifying ways to prevent the factors you have discovered from contributing to another error. Some of the solutions may involve education and practice in critical thinking—others may be systems or management strategies.

10. Every time we do a root cause analysis on a sentinel event I realize that some nurses don't recognize it when things don't make sense—such as when a nurse gave 80 mEq of KCl to a patient with renal problems 3 times a day for 2 days. How can we prevent this kind of mistake?

This example certainly underscores the need for clinical judgment. Asking "What's wrong with this picture?" can prevent or catch errors. Some nurses do seem to shun responsibility for questioning orders. Maybe the dose in the example was intended by the prescriber to be 8.0. The zero trailing the decimal point is a culprit in many medication errors.

Questioning is an important part of critical thinking and an essential part of safe practice. Questioning physician orders is an opportunity for the nurse to gain greater respect from physician and pharmacist colleagues and to learn as well.

In the example, the nurse evidenced a lack of knowledge—about potassium and about patients with renal problems—and failure to monitor patient response adequately if this went on for two days. It's important to remember that critical thinking operates on a knowledge base. Nurses need access to information and must be expected to refer to credible sources of information.

11. How can I create a performance improvement plan for a nurse who just can't seem to think?

Begin by presenting the evidence that the nurse can't seem to think. Presenting the evidence has a punitive, courtroom drama ring to it. That is not the concept of presenting evidence that I'm emphasizing. Critical thinking involves assembling evidence to support conclusions—in this case, the conclusion that this nurse just can't think. When you begin to assemble evidence, you may come to alternative or additional conclusions.

However, when you have identified the evidence, you will have identified specific problems to address with performance expectations. Is the nurse failing to collect sufficient information? Is the nurse lacking in the needed knowledge base? Is the nurse having difficulty asserting and asking questions? A performance improvement plan cannot succeed unless it contains specific improvements required and specific evidence of the desired improvement. The manager must also clarify the expectations as needed until the manager and nurse reach a mutual understanding of the terms of the plan.

12. When I think about using critical thinking in appraising staff performance, I have to admit that I think of criticizing performance. How does critical thinking fit with positive appraisals of performance?

Critique is a key critical thinking skill. Remember that critique identifies and celebrates strengths as well as weaknesses. In fact, the atmosphere that sustains critical thinking needs to include rewards for thinking.

As Henry Ford said, "Thinking is work, which is the probable reason why so few people engage in it." Nurses face so many challenges every day! To demand that they also challenge the rules, question orders, ask "What's wrong with this picture?" and otherwise demonstrate critical thinking can feel overwhelming and beyond the nurses' capabilities.

When nurses experience positive feedback for their critical thinking and encouragement to support each other as critical thinkers, critical thinking flourishes. Remember the management maxim, "What gets measured gets produced; What gets rewarded gets produced again." The manager's critical thinking comes into play in offering meaningful rewards and giving positive feedback that goes beyond saying, "Nice job," to saying "Great work with Mrs. Jones.

By catching the potential for drug-drug interaction in her medication profile you saved her from discomfort and from danger of a bleed. You're really an asset to our team." In the latter response, the manager predicts and recognizes the effect of the nurse's action.

13. What about the medical departments and the other clinical departments? How can I get them on board with the efforts in the Nursing Department to improve clinical judgment and critical thinking?

What are the patient care issues that these other departments are facing? Find out and, in fact, make a habit of finding out on an ongoing basis. That kind of attitude of inquiry fuels critical thinking and can serve as the basis for interdisciplinary efforts to improve care.

Identify the critical thinking strategies that address other departments' issues and share your thoughts with them—at every level:

- During bedside interactions between nursing staff and members of other disciplines
- During interactions between nurse managers and members of other disciplines
- During nursing representation on all of the interdepartmental committees:
  - Quality/organizational performance
  - Nursing/pharmacy
  - New products
  - Materials management
  - Other committees and task forces
- During nursing director representation in medical department meetings

If you have adopted or adapted a particular critical thinking model, share it with colleagues in other disciplines—not as a graphic image, but as an approach or perhaps as a series of questions to ask in clinical situations.

14. Aren't clinical judgment and critical thinking really the province of RNs? Do you think that UAP really ought to be expected to do these things?

Well-defined protocols guide much of the work of UAP. However, UAP also face situations that protocols do not define. For example,

- How to respond to a patient's question or complaint
- Whether and when to report unanticipated findings to the RN

During training and orientation, UAP need to practice their judgment skills in response to scenarios that are within their scope of practice. We can expect UAP to think critically about basic issues such as safety and infection control. Expecting them to think critically does not mean that we need to supply them with elaborate rationales or the knowledge base of the RN. But we can expect them to question unexpected findings—not simply record the finding and report it to the RN at the end of the shift. UAP can examine the assumptions they make to ensure that those assumptions hold true in a given situation. UAP can recognize opportunities to safely implement alternative approaches, such as alternative feeding techniques if conventional methods are not effective. Boundaries and knowledge base for UAP critical thinking differ from expectations for RN critical thinking. Communicate these expectations clearly to UAP.

After all, elementary school curricula now teach critical thinking strategies. If young children can learn to think critically about issues within the scope of their knowledge and roles, adults who are giving direct patient care can certainly be expected to think critically.

Remember that unlicensed caregivers also include patients, their family, and friends who participate in care. Include critical thinking strategies in patient/family teaching as well. Use scenarios. Let them identify circumstances that would require a call to the health professional. Help them learn to recognize "What's wrong with this picture?" in time to prevent a risk situation or an exacerbation of illness.

15. Even if we expect UAP do so some critical thinking and use some judgment do you really believe that non-clinical departments can relate to critical thinking?

I hope so! I hope that the security officers analyze situations that may pose threats to security. I hope they maintain a skeptical attitude toward suspicious behavior and investigate. I hope dietary workers don't assume that newly delivered food is fresh even though it smells funny. Continue on this trip around the organization from finance to human resources to volunteer services and throughout the entire organization. You cannot escape the conclusion that quality of care, safety, cost-effectiveness, and every other aspect of the organization's performance can improve with alert staff asking "What's wrong with this picture?" or "What could be improved?" and employing other critical thinking strategies to identify and solve problems.

But this can occur only when critical thinking is effectively translated in terms meaningful to staff at various levels and in various departments. It's a situation reminiscent of the emphasis on vision, mission, and values a number of years ago. Organizations that succeeded in bringing those ideas to life assisted staff of all departments at all levels to interpret vision, mission, and values specifically in their own roles.

16. Why not just use a standardized test to screen for and validate critical thinking competency?

Because you will not find a test that is valid for the purpose of assuring that nurses think critically in practice. Critical thinking defies measurement with a single objective test. It is true that there are standardized tests available that purport to measure critical thinking and some of them do measure selected critical thinking behaviors and attitudes. However, objective tests do not require the test taker to generate an answer—only to select an answer from a limited number of choices. As Dorothy del Bueno (1990) wrote, "Unfortunately patients seldom present nurses with four possible options to solve their health-care problems" (p. 6). And even if tests include some short answer questions, there are probably important uses of critical thinking and clinical judgment in your setting that the test will miss.

The most valid way to test critical thinking competency is to identify what critical thinking looks like in your setting, present sample situations to staff members, and ask how they will handle those situations. Of course you still face the limitation that people will not always behave the way they state that they will on a test. You also need to think through the model answers and identify which elements of those answers are essential criteria. Then ensure that critical thinking and clinical judgment are expected in practice and evaluated in the performance appraisal process.

17. Why don't they teach the nurses to think critically in nursing school? It seems to me it's all up to us in the practice setting. For what are the schools accountable?

Many nurses in practice seem astonished to learn that critical thinking *is* a major emphasis in schools of nursing. In fact, accrediting bodies have required schools of nursing to document their teaching and measuring of critical thinking.

Schools are accountable for preparing graduates to *enter* nursing practice. In my opinion that means that schools are accountable for ensuring that graduates have mastered the critical thinking skills and attitudes they need to practice at the entry level. For example:

- I expect a new graduate to ask lots of questions—to identify what he/she knows, needs to find out, and what will be a credible source of needed information.
- I expect new graduates to think-out-loud with preceptors and tell the preceptor how they have reached a conclusion or decision so that the preceptor can offer some feedback.
- I expect new graduates to accept accountability for their own practice—and that includes entry level critical thinking about clinical situations.

18. Why can't staff development use orientation to screen out the nurses who don't think critically?

Staff development educators would ask you why managers and others who interview can't screen them out before they even get to orientation. Managers and staff development specialists need to collaborate closely and continuously to eliminate any "disconnects" between what goes on in orientation and what is expected on the clinical unit. In the orientation process, offer opportunities for orientees to demonstrate and validate their critical thinking skills. Ask them to compare the policies and procedures of their new employer with past experience. Ask for their responses to patient care situations that commonly occur. When the staff development specialist identifies weaknesses in critical thinking, he/she needs to share those concerns with the appropriate manager—that is, give feedback that describes the nurse's response—rather than labeling the nurse as a poor critical thinker. Experienced staff development specialists become quite astute at identifying orientees who are at risk for failure and dissatisfaction. A critical thinking challenge for the staff development specialist is to define the criteria that are used when making these often intuitive judgments. Those criteria might inform some improved screening practices.

19. Isn't expecting preceptors to deal with critical thinking just too much to expect?

Not if you perceive critical thinking as a *way* of going about patient care rather than more items on the already voluminous competency checklist. Preceptors display their own critical thinking when they think out loud with orientees, making their own clinical judgment visible. If such monologue is not appropriate in the patient's presence, the preceptor can alert the orientee to particular aspects that they will discuss in detail at a later time. The preceptor can also:

- Expect the orientee to think out loud. This process alone will sharpen the critical thinking skills of both parties.

- Engage the orientee in a compare-and-contrast exercise, asking the orientee to identify similarities and differences with the orientee's previous experience.
- Ask plenty of open-ended questions: "What else do you need to know?" "Where can you find that information?"
- Keep the attitude of inquiry continuously alive through the relationship with the orientee—including identifying and clarifying ways to make the preceptorship more effective for both parties.

20. Would it work to do critical thinking education in annual mandatory education?

Annual mandatory education can certainly include opportunities for staff to demonstrate critical thinking skills. Consider setting up simulated situations—with actual equipment, pictures, audiotape or videotape. Ask the staff what is wrong (or right, or what could be improved) in that picture. That's a practical and realistic way to get staff thinking about real safety issues rather than simply watching a film festival or reciting acronyms. If you have endorsed and implemented a particular critical thinking model, question, or other hallmark for critical thinking efforts, annual mandatory education is an appropriate time to ensure that staff are on board with the program.

21. I'm in staff development and my boss says I need to set up a 30-minute critical thinking inservice class for all shifts—what's the best way to use the time?

First get the boss to be explicit about what he/she has in mind as the outcome of this intensive foray into critical thinking. Clarify the boss's expectations and define the outcomes that you can realistically accomplish. You might want to reconsider the 30-minute inservice class on all shifts—is that really the best way to accomplish the goal?

22. What kinds of critical thinking education can I expect from the staff development department?

One of my favorite critical thinking techniques is to turn the question around. That is, you're asking what you can expect. Turn that question around and challenge yourself to specify what you think you need. What outcomes would you expect from staff development support of clinical judgment and critical thinking?

Like every other department in the facility, the staff development department is challenged to respond to needs for its services. The most effective way to work with staff development is to work collaboratively. The staff development effort is most likely to succeed when it addresses particular, specific practice outcomes. For example, if you enter collaboration with the staff development specialist by identifying the need for nurses to question and clarify medication orders more frequently, you will be more likely to experience success with the outcome and a satisfying process than if you request that the staff development specialist teach the nurses to think critically.

Also, like other departments, staff development sets priorities. The promise of measurable improvements in patient safety and patient care usually helps requests to ascend higher on the priority list. The nursing unit should collaborate with the staff development specialist to identify ways in which the unit can supply evidence that staff development efforts have succeeded. Look for evidence that is readily available in records and does not require additional means and procedures for collecting data.

As an aside—try turning questions around to stimulate the thinking of the person who asks you a question. Obviously that's not an appropriate technique for all questions asked of you—for example, when patients ask for information you will usually simply provide the information rather than engage in a Socratic dialogue. Even with patients though, if some of their questions require that they apply information you have taught in patient teaching, you will be empowering the patient for self-care when you ask questions that will help the patient learn to apply knowledge about his/her disease and treatment.

RESOURCES

Case, B. (1994). Walking around the elephant: A critical thinking strategy for problem solving. *The Journal of Continuing Education in Nursing, 25*(3), 101–109.

Case, B. (1999). Manager as infusion pump: Facilitating continuous flow of critical thinking in the nursing department. *Advance for Nurses, 17*(1), 16–17.

Case, B. (1999). *Preceptor workbook: Advanced practice nurse.* Chicago, IL: Loyola University of Chicago Marcella Niehoff School of Nursing.

Case, B. (2000). *Critical thinking: Addressing staffing issues.* San Diego: Professional Development Center of American Mobile Healthcare (**www.rn.com**).

del Bueno, D. (1990). Evaluation: Myths, mysteries and obsessions. *Journal of Nursing Administration, 20*(11), 4–7.

Hansten, R., & Washburn, M. (1999). Individual and organizational accountability for development of critical thinking. *Journal of Nursing Administration, 29*(11), 39–45.

Paul, R. (1995). *Critical thinking: How to prepare students for a rapidly changing world.* Santa Rosa, CA: Foundation for Critical Thinking.

Chapter 12: Setting Priorities

"At all events, one may safely say, a nurse cannot be with the patient, open the door, eat her meals, take a message, all at one and the same time. Nevertheless the person in charge seems to look the impossibility in the face."

—Florence Nightingale

1. I feel as if I'm constantly being challenged to readjust my priorities. How can I set some priorities that have some staying power?

Steven Covey (1989) recommended a solid approach to this challenge. He first reminded us that each of us has a "true north." By this he means that we each have core values, a personal mission, and a philosophy. We may not yet have articulated those guides to our lives and if we have not, doing so is a first step toward tackling the matter of priorities. He suggested that once we have a clear sense of direction in our lives (metaphorically, the true north of the compass) we can strive to align our priorities consistent with our true north.

These ideas may seem a little esoteric for the pace of a busy nursing unit. However, you do have personal/professional values and a philosophy of life and nursing—whether or not you have clearly articulated them. It is hoped that you have chosen a work setting consistent with your own values. If you have not, and cannot resolve the differences, you may need to seek a work setting more in concert with your values.

Covey suggested that we can classify all of our activities on two dimensions:

• Urgency
• Importance

Obviously on the nursing unit, urgent and important demands take precedence—life-threatening situations or high-risk situations need our first attention. But Covey cautioned that situations that seem urgent (for example, because a frustrated MD is acting out) are not necessarily more important than some less urgent concerns, such as reassuring a quietly anxious patient. He urged us to avoid letting squeaky-wheels or sacred cow habits and routines distract us from more important matters.

Critical thinking is essential to sort out urgency and importance. As you consider the activities you must prioritize, think about how urgent each really is—When must this be dealt with? In the next five minutes? The next hour? Before the end of the shift? On the next shift? Tomorrow okay? Before discharge?

Critical thinking and clinical judgment are essential because sometimes urgency is dictated by usual hospital routines. Routines preserve order, standardize, and ensure safety. But there are occasions when other needs are more important than routines.

The priorities that have staying power are long-term priorities connected solidly to your professional values. View daily priority setting in the context of how daily priorities build toward and give life to your professional values and philosophy.

2. All problems seem to be urgent and important. Do all problems need immediate attention?

The opportunities for critical thinking that we uncovered do not all need immediate attention. Life threatening and risk situations obviously must be addressed promptly. Other situations in need of improvement may be matters that can be addressed with a policy change, with changing unlicensed assistive personnel (UAP) assignments or taking other actions. Guard against losing those latter opportunities just because they can't be addressed today. Channel those needs and suggestions to the proper person—the charge nurse, the nurse manager or other appropriate person. Nurses become highly skilled at working effectively around difficulties and less than optimal situations. But when nurses continue to "make do" on a daily basis, the potential for improving the system is lost.

3. With all of the mandated education, accreditation compliance issues, and administration's flavor-of-the-month initiatives, how can we possibly give priority to clinical judgment and critical thinking?

How can you not? How else will you survive the challenges you are mentioning? Critical thinking produces creative solutions within given parameters or a given context. That's what differentiates critical thinking from unbridled creativity.

All of the challenges you mentioned have interdisciplinary implications. Effective plans for mandated education, accreditation compliance, and most administrative directives require that you elicit the perspectives of the different parties and disciplines involved. That means first that each party defines the problem from his/her own point of view and identifies what the solution needs to contain in order to work for him/her. That kind of analysis and collaboration is an interpersonal form of critical thinking.

Remember that critical thinking is a way of doing things—not another thing to do. It takes a little longer to be deliberate, to analyze, to elicit perspectives, and to consider a variety of approaches. But the approach is more likely to work and to endure—especially when the decision is one that affects many different units, disciplines, or parties. You recapture the investment of time you make on the front end by avoiding the need to return to problems again and again. Ineffective solutions often result when you solve the wrong problem or fail to consider all the relevant perspectives.

4. How does critical thinking relate to some of our clinical priority-setting approaches?

First of all, it's important to recognize that we encounter situations that are *not* opportunities for critical thinking. True emergencies and many high-risk, urgent situations call for immediate response—often protocol-driven. The protocols of course are the result of previous critical thinking and experimentation. Critical thinking comes into play in recognizing what's wrong with the picture and that a protocol is indicated. But once a protocol is put into effect, there is usually little deviation or consideration of a variety of alternatives.

Sometimes, however, we eliminate more situations than we should from the list of critical thinking opportunities. For example, we sometimes take for granted that the policy and procedure for some aspect of practice is the only way to manage that situation. Certainly we need to abide by policies and procedures as long as we have them on the books. But, we need also to be open to recognizing the need to alter a policy and procedure or consider alternatives.

There's a parallel between conventional ABC (airway, breathing, circulation) priority setting and using critical thinking. Airway is first because breathing can occur only when an airway is established and circulation doesn't accomplish anything without oxygenated blood. The critical thinking "airway" comprises the first questions we ask—when we recognize that there is something wrong with the picture or that a situation can be improved. But that first level of questions is only a pathway into the situation. We have to keep more specific questions coming and the answers forthcoming (as in breathing in and out) until we have stabilized the situation. And simultaneously, we have to keep the questions, answers, and actions they suggest circulating around the situation until we achieve the desired outcome. And then we have to check vital signs from time to time (how frequently depends upon the stability of the situation) to be sure the solution still works.

So in terms of daily priority setting, we have to have a plan, but remain constantly alert for compromised airways—that is, for what's wrong with this picture? And be ready to resuscitate when we encounter the clinical picture with something wrong, something at risk, or something that we can improve.

5. Where do we start to tackle deficits in clinical judgment and critical thinking?

How are you identifying these deficits? If you identify lapses in clinical judgment and critical thinking, you must be looking at more than a result like a patient fall, a patient complaint, or some other negative outcome. You evidently know or suspect that someone failed to think critically or use sound judgment.

Maybe a fall resulted when a patient who was not otherwise at risk for falling took a newly prescribed drug with powerful hypotensive effect. Maybe a patient complained because the nurse awakened him for a routine blood pressure when he had just dozed off after an agitated, sleepless night. In both of these examples, the nurse either lacked an important piece of information, or neglected to incorporate a piece of information and deviate from routine procedure based upon that knowledge.

Most often the negative outcome comes to light first, and then in reconstructing the process that led to the outcome, lapses in thinking or judgment become evident. Occasionally you observe a nurse about to act with flawed judgment or thinking and have the opportunity to intervene in time to prevent the negative outcome—a near miss instead of a mistake.

Start improving judgment and thinking at the point at which you identify the lapse. In other words, if a negative outcome alerts you, start backtracking through the process that led to the outcome. If you intervene and prevent a negative outcome, backtrack from this near-miss to find out where judgment or thinking broke down.

When you engage in this process you are really applying your own critical thinking. You are analyzing the process that led to an outcome. Further, you apply critical thinking skills by searching for alternatives that can prevent the lapse of judgment or thinking in the future. For example, the nurse did not take fall precautions and the patient fell after taking the powerful hypotensive drug. Why did this occur? Because the nurse did not know the effect of the drug? Or, because the nurse had just come on duty and because of a failure in communication did not know that the patient was receiving a new drug? There may be other explanations as well. With only these two possibilities, you can see that each cause leads to different preventive actions.

Make a habit of analyzing negative outcomes and near miss situations. Encourage others to do the same. In addition to correcting and preventing the deficit in a particular situation, the process will have a ripple effect. You will identify other situations to which the preventive strategy applies and you will be building critical thinking skills through practice.

6. What is the dissatisfaction/effort model for setting priorities?

The dissatisfaction/effort model offers a priority setting model that you can use as an individual or with a group for priority setting. One benefit of using the model with a group is that the model makes visible the ways in which priorities of individuals differ from priorities for the group. In addition to building consensus on priorities, individuals can take ownership of those matters of individual priority.

Here's how it works as a group effort:

1. Brainstorm with the staff. In the nonjudgmental atmosphere of brainstorming, identify all of the issues that you consider potential priorities for the group.

2. Take the critical thinking approach to brainstorming by asking the question, "What else?" when you think you have completed the comprehensive list of issues. If you force yourselves to remain quiet until you add at least one more issue to the "exhaustive" list, you will often find that those last ideas are particularly creative and worthwhile.

3. As individuals, each group member rates each item on two dimensions:

   a. Dissatisfaction—On a scale of 1–10, how dissatisfied are you with the present status of this particular issue? If the item is something that you currently lack, for example a self-staffing model, the question is: How dissatisfied are you that you do not have such a model?

   b. Effort—On a scale of 1–10, how much effort are you willing to expend addressing this issue?

4. Average the ratings of the group members so that you arrive at an average dissatisfaction score and an average effort score for each issue.

5. Now comes the fun part: plotting the items on a grid (see Figure 12-1).

Each issue has both a dissatisfaction score and a commitment of effort score. Using these scores as coordinates, plot each issue on the grid.

The example shows the plotting (X) of 4 of 30 issues identified by the nursing staff of a critical care unit.

- ACLS Course = Dissatisfaction 2;
- Commitment of Effort 10

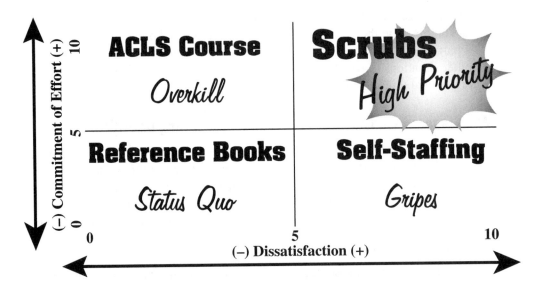

Figure 12-1: The Dissatisfaction/Effort Model—Priorities Grid

- Reference Books = Dissatisfaction 3;
- Commitment of Effort 3
- Self-Staffing = Dissatisfaction 8;
- Commitment of Effort 4
- Scrubs = Dissatisfaction 8;
- Commitment of Effort 10

Since the staff is quite satisfied with the ACLS Course, even though they are willing to commit effort to improving it, to do so would be overkill. The staff is quite satisfied with the unit reference books and not willing to invest effort in identifying new ones and using unit funds to purchase them. Therefore, the reference books can remain status quo. The staff is very dissatisfied with the lack of a self-staffing plan; however, they are not willing to invest effort to create a plan. So, self-staffing is a gripe. The staff is very dissatisfied with the lack of scrubs purchased with unit funds and very willing to invest effort in selecting and purchasing unit-specific scrub uniforms. So scrubs emerges as a high priority.

Note that the use of average scores gives an indication of the priorities *for the group as a whole.* Any issue may be of high priority to some individual even though the group on average does not rate it high. In this example, there may be one or two staff members who are willing to invest effort in creating a self-

staffing plan. Those two individuals might volunteer to draft a plan which probably the group would support since they are dissatisfied that they lack such a plan.

To avoid the calculation of average scores, a simple high, moderate or low rating could be given to each issue instead of a numerical score.

7. Is there a way to integrate critical thinking strategies with other priorities?

Critical thinking integrates beautifully with other priorities because critical
thinking is a *way* of doing things—not an additional thing to do. Just be sure to
make the critical thinking process evident. For example, make a point of verbalizing your thought processes as you:

- Reflect on your progress toward accomplishing your priorities
- Critique your priority setting
- Ask plenty of questions as you address each priority
- Seek the perspectives of relevant others
- Collaborate
- Assemble evidence to support your actions

8. Can't we just give the nurses a specific step-wise critical thinking process to follow—like nursing process?

In a word, "No." Probably that one word answer is not very satisfying and that
illustrates the value of asking questions that require more than a yes or no
answer. When you require more than yes or no, you are asking the other party to
make his/her reasoning visible to you.

So, to elaborate: Critical thinking is not a step-wise process. You can certainly
use a model or a series of questions as a guide for critical thinking. Some applications of critical thinking such as making nursing diagnoses, evaluating a
patient's status and response to treatment, and analyzing certain kinds of data
do have a sequence of steps. But critical thinking is bigger than a series of
steps. Critical thinking comprises many strategies, behaviors, and attitudes that
often overlap.

Critical thinking has both a logical and a creative dimension. I like to represent
critical thinking as a light bulb—the universal symbol for new ideas. But a special kind of light bulb—a light bulb which has a question mark as a filament.
The question mark symbolizes the attitude of inquiry that drives critical thinking and the logical process.

Critical thinking requires a very sophisticated type of creativity. Solutions arrived at through critical thinking fit defined parameters or criteria. Some of the biggest creative challenges in nursing are made challenging by the number of criteria that must be satisfied. For example, devising an effective discharge plan for a patient who has multiple co-morbidities and care needs; creating safe and equitable patient assignments in tight staffing situations; or managing your time during a shift with lots of unexpected events such as admissions, dramatic changes in patients' conditions or systems failures involving computer systems, pharmacy, and other departments.

9. How can we keep critical thinking a priority? It seems like our usual approach is to identify a problem, do an inservice class, and check it off the list.

If that is truly the approach you are taking, I'll bet that many of those problems reappear on the list in no time. One of the ways in which critical thinking differs from problem solving is in the emphasis on examining a problem carefully before hurrying to solve it. Consider different definitions of the problem. Sometimes we solve the wrong problem. Did you ever change a policy to solve a problem only to find that once you implemented the policy the annoying symptoms of the problem persisted? Take the time to define and redefine the problem. Incorporate other perspectives than your own into the problem definition.

Another difference in emphasis between critical thinking and problem solving is that in critical thinking we make a point of rechecking at intervals to ensure that the solution we chose continues to be valid despite changing circumstances.

Remember that you can never stand in the same river twice. Different water flows past every instant; perhaps the course of the river or the riverbed changes and, of course, you yourself change over time. So it is important as a critical thinker to verify that a solution still works given changes and new information that may now be available.

A final comment on the inservice education "fix." Inservice education, or any educational effort for that matter, has little influence on outcomes unless management supports the effort and expects nurses to practice what they learned. One piece of critical thinking that we all master pretty well is identifying our boss's priorities. The management maxim, "Expect it, or forget it," applies. What the manager focuses on and rewards is what the staff will produce—no matter what they learned in the inservice class.

Staff development specialists and nurse managers share the accountability for collaborating, monitoring, and giving feedback to each other about what is communicated in educational offerings and how effectively the effort has addressed the intended outcome. If it's working, both need to reflect on how they succeeded together in order to make a habit of such effective collaboration. And if it's not, both need to reflect on why not and relish the opportunity to improve.

If you seem to be addressing problems "by the ones," you need to aim beyond the technique to fix an individual problem. Instead, aim for a strategy to prevent related problems and recurrence of this one. James Carville and Paul Begala (2002) related a metaphor to illustrate the difference between technique and strategy. They wrote that a lion can barely get enough calories to survive by capturing and eating field mice all day long. If the lion bags an antelope, that kill will feed the pride of lions. But to get the antelope, the lion must stop pouncing on mice and come up with a strategy and tactics.

10. As an organization it seems that departments and units have different priorities. I'm not even sure that the members of my staff share similar priorities. How do we pick a focus?

One model that works nicely for priority setting with a group is described in my response to question 5.

Individual staff members will surely have differing priorities. However, all need to endorse the goals of the organization and the unit. At the unit level, the manager needs to communicate what organizational and unit goals look like in daily actions. Also, at the unit level, when staff members participate in setting priorities, they are more likely to endorse them actively.

Departments and units will differ in priorities because their roles in the organization differ. It is hoped that all of these priorities and roles support broad goals of safe, effective, high quality patient care.

Rather than seeking consensus on all priorities, the critical thinking approach is to clarify the differences in perspectives—for example, to help the ICU nurses understand why it is so important to the ED nurses to get the critical patients into the ICU and out of the ED and to help the ED nurses understand what has to happen in order to clear a bed. Understanding one another's viewpoint will not solve the problem or relieve the frustration. However, it may help identify who needs to get involved and in what ways in order to fix the current situation to the extent possible—even more importantly to prevent ongoing recurrences of the same problem.

A reasonable and constructive focus might be to identify approaches that meet the needs of all of the relevant players' perspectives on any given issue.

11. We have some organizational priorities. The executive group sets them in their annual retreat. Most of them don't relate to me and the unit. Do I need different priorities for the unit?

The executive group has failed you if they have not provided the direction you need to connect with the organizational priorities they identified. Sometimes designers of organizational priorities draft sweeping statements in global terms intending to encompass activities in every segment of the organization. But the result lacks the specificity that managers need to align their operations with organizational priorities.

Ask your direct supervisor what these organizational priorities imply for your daily operations. This is not a time to make creative guesses about what terms like "vertical integration" mean to the unit. Whatever *you* think the framers of these priorities had in mind, the executive who evaluates your performance and the unit's performance will be using the definition *he/she* had in mind.

It is not reasonable to expect the executive to lay out a detailed plan about what the priorities mean for your daily operations—that is your job and it will require some critical thinking. But, if no connection is apparent to you, you need and deserve some guidance to help you align your priorities with organizational goals.

12. Are there some critical thinking approaches that I can use to organize my day more effectively?

By asking that question you're indicating that you see a need for improvement—that you are not satisfied with the way you have been organizing your day. That is a good place to start with the critical thinking technique of reflecting. In what ways is your current method of organizing your day failing you? That critical thinking question will lead you to a more productive, satisfying day if you act on the answers you discover.

Do you set such ambitious daily goals that you set yourself up to fail? Analyze some of these goals to break them into manageable pieces. Maybe you've had "Nursing Documentation Chart Audits" on your list for two weeks. You've got the audit form and the plan is to review open records. You're just not finding the time to do it. If you put one chart per day on the list could you get that done? Could you cease and desist from all other activities during the last 20 minutes of the work day and review a record?

Develop the habit of using a verb to state each item on your daily list. That is, articulate what you plan to *do* about it. So the item on today's list is not

"Staffing budget." Instead it is, "Analyze last year's overtime and agency costs." Let ensuing days' lists include other specific daily steps toward completing the staffing budget.

13. Sounds great, but I have more than I can do in a day, no matter how well I prioritize. Can critical thinking help me get more done?

Maybe what you have set out to accomplish in a day is more appropriate for a week. Perhaps you can make some progress on each item every day—or perhaps make each item a major focus of a day.

Look at the responses to questions 1 and 6 in this chapter. Are you letting urgent matters overtake important matters on your priority list (question 1)? Are you expending energies on overkill or status quo items (question 6)?

Perhaps you believe that you have so much going on that you are always working on a number of goals at the same time (personal and family-related goals included). Consequently, you are not satisfied with accomplishments in any realm. What can you do differently, or not at all? What can you delegate to others in your professional and personal world? How can you better focus your attention?

Different individuals will discover different needs for improvement in their individual methods of getting organized. Oftentimes seeking some input from another person's perspective will offer just the insight you need to make a positive change in organizing your day. And even though you view your own planning as needing improvement, you may have some constructive suggestions for someone else.

Whatever you learn by reflecting on your current system, commit to taking action. Do just one thing differently. Reflect on the results—did it work? Would it work if you got up earlier? Or had lunch at a different time? Or modified something else? Or do you need to abandon that approach and try something different? The point is to try small adjustments until you have a plan that is more satisfying.

You cannot hope to succeed without a plan for the day. Create your plan before the day begins—before you leave work on the previous day, or during your commute to work. If you think you don't have time to make a plan, you definitely need to rethink.

A plan allows you to experience a sense of control. When you have a plan you equip yourself for the unexpected. You have a clear picture of what you plan to accomplish. When other demands arise, you can see immediately what you must do to accommodate the new demands. Defer the new demands until tomorrow? Delegate something that is on today's list? Move something on today's list to tomorrow, or to next week?

You are the only one who has the power to organize your day and control your response to the day's events. Reframe the discouraged, frustrated, over-whelmed or even desperate thoughts and feelings that arise from a sense of dis-organization. Take control with a plan and a reflective approach toward improving it continuously.

14. How can I really say that critical thinking has any impact on our goals and priorities?

Critical thinking is a process. To give critical thinking its due as a contributor to achieving goals, analyze the process that led to successes—you may also dis-cover breakdowns in critical thinking that interfered with your success. For example, you may have fallen short of a goal because you failed to identify all of the relevant stakeholders and incorporate their perspectives. On the other hand, you may attribute some success to critical thinking if on the road to suc-cessfully achieving a goal, you questioned your assumptions about the way you have traditionally provided care.

Results alone cannot reveal if or how critical thinking contributed to success. Analyzing the process gives you some practice with critical thinking as well as giving you a way to make the benefits of critical thinking explicit.

15. I think using good clinical judgment is always the number one priority. It's a huge safety issue. Is there any other way to address it in a bigger picture than a case-by-case "What went wrong?"?

A case-by-case "What went wrong?" isn't a bad place to start. But, let it lead you somewhere. Too often examining mistakes, incidents or unusual occur-rences goes no further than identifying the problem and assigning the blame.

Do you see any themes in these situations? Are nurses distracted? If so why and how can you fix it? Admonishing the nurses to "Just say no," to distractions will not work.

Re-examine the approaches you have put in place to prevent recurrences. Sometimes we forget to notice the negative instance and congratulate ourselves for the absence of a problem. For example, suppose you began storing the two concentrations of IV heparin on separate shelves in the medication room because the similar appearance of the bags had contributed to errors and near misses. Track the result of the change and celebrate the improvement in safety. However, if you maintain the same rate of errors and near misses, there is another dragon to flush out and slay.

Have periodic time-limited safety alerts. For a specified time period, such as one week, ask staff to be alert for safety risks in unit practices and in the environment. Collect the staff's observations on rounds, in report, or with some structure similar to a suggestion box. Look for themes in the risks identified. Create and implement action plans to improve safety. The periodic focus may help improve safety awareness on an ongoing basis.

16. We have some much higher priorities than critical thinking! These nurses don't know how to delegate and we're always in a staffing crisis. Doesn't critical thinking belong a little lower on the priority list than some of these other issues?

Critical thinking belongs in the thick of those priorities you mention. Critical thinking approaches can help manage delegation and staffing challenges. In both cases, the critical thinking process begins with discerning what is wrong with the picture. Why aren't the nurses delegating? What is causing the staffing crisis?

Recognize that the whole of the problem with delegating is *not* a cognitive one. That is, it is just as much about the RNs' level of trust and confidence in the competence of LPNs and UAP as it is about the skill of delegating.

Get some feedback from the nurses about why they are not delegating appropriately. Do they lack confidence in the competence of their assistants? If so, how can they build confidence? Do they need to observe the LPNs and UAP in action? Do the LPNs and/or UAP have need for further training or practice with selected skills? When the RNs fail to delegate, their assistants do not get opportunities to practice and retain the skills they learned in training.

Use a resource such as those recommended in the resources for this chapter to coach the nurses in delegation in response to the needs you identify. First the RN must gain a clear understanding of the competencies of assistive personnel and confidence in the competence of those individuals.

17. How does critical thinking help with the process of delegation?

Effective delegation requires critical thinking. The RN makes a judgment about the stability of each patient and delegates accordingly. This is a different approach than assigning all the baths to UAP—some baths are more appropriately reserved for the RN; for example, an unstable patient, or a patient at risk for skin breakdown who needs a complete assessment. If the RN determines that some baths require RN skill, then what other tasks can UAP perform with these particular patients on this particular shift?

There are probably numerous factors contributing to staffing crises: vacancies, sick calls, patient acuity, patient turnover, and others. The manager needs to rise to the occasion with critical thinking skills: analyze the contributing factors and try some approaches to address the causes. If the manager responds only by calling all off-duty staff to fill staffing holes, or resorting to temporary agency nurses on a shift-by-shift basis, the staffing crises will occur regularly.

But, while the manager is getting to the root of the problem and trying to improve the future staffing picture, the immediate staffing shortage needs attention. Part of the answer may lie in a true critical thinking approach to delegation, the beginnings of which are suggested above. When all staff members contribute their skills in the most effective fashion, staffing crises can be avoided.

When staffing is less than optimal, nurses need to think critically about priorities for specific patients and for the given shift. Within the policies and procedures of the facility, and with proper consultation and support, the nurses need the freedom to make professional decisions about what usual routine activities can be deferred.

Deciding what can be "left out" on a given shift requires sound clinical judgment. It is not as simple as dictating "no baths," or "no linen changes." The nurse decides based on individual patient needs and unit needs within the context of the particular shift.

If policies and procedures don't permit nurses enough autonomy, or if nurses lack the expertise to make those judgments, those too are issues that need to be addressed.

You'll find some additional suggestions for short staffing situations in response to the next question.

18. When we're short staffed, I get concerned about patient safety and so does the staff. Are there any strategies that can help us feel more confident at those times?

A very important one is to recognize that critical thinking is at risk in short-staffing situations. Be aware that the frenzy of a short-staffed shift can narrow your perspective and dull your sensitivity to subtle clues that a patient may be at risk.

Especially when staffing is less than optimal, begin the shift by identifying the potential safety risks with each patient and ensure that you make rounds to assess the status of the patient vis-à-vis those risks at least every hour and more frequently if safety requires it. Depending upon the situation, it may be safe to delegate certain of those periodic safety risk checks to a UAP.

19. **There's a lot of variation in the experience of the staff. How can I help them set and achieve individual priorities for performance improvement and job satisfaction?**

First of all, recognize and celebrate those experience differences. One key to job satisfaction lies in respecting each others' perspectives and learning from each other.

You may wonder what a 30-year veteran has to learn from a 30-day-old grad. The 30-day-old grad takes a naive perspective on much of what goes on in the nursing unit. In a critical thinking atmosphere which welcomes questions and multiple perspectives, the new grad can get clarification and information. However, the more seasoned nurses need to suspend their judgment on some of the naive comments of the neophyte. Most often, the new grad's question simply requires an informative answer. But sometimes the new grad's question, "Why do you do it that way?" or "Why is that important?" or "What if you . . ?" can shatter some assumptions about "the way we do things here," and lead to improvements in care.

The career development aspect of the new grad's job is to gain competence and identify the parts of nursing that offer the greatest joy to the individual. That requires the new grad to reflect frequently on his/her experience and learning needs.

Sometimes nurses characterized as "many points between those extremes" (of the nurse with 30 years of experience and the new graduate of 30 days ago) feel neglected. They don't enjoy the benefits and respect of senior staff, nor do they receive the special treatment reserved for new graduates. They may be among those most eager for new learning and new opportunities since they have mastered the basics of the specialty and have many more potentially productive years on the staff.

Look for ways to help the senior staff members achieve the developmental task of generativity. It may be in contributing to new staff members or it may be in contributing to patients or to the unit in special ways. Help seasoned staff raise questions such as, "What could be improved here?" "What has bugged me about working here for the 25 years I've been on staff?" "When patients return to the unit, what do they tell us could have better helped them to manage on their own after last discharged from the hospital?" Is there a way to pilot test some approaches in answer to those questions?

Although I am responding to the question you asked about individual priorities, it is important to remember that constructive working relationships, team work, and some unit goals that all endorse are vital to job satisfaction and nurse retention.

20. I think the nurses on my staff are just burning out left and right. They just want to get through the shift. How can I possibly get them to see critical thinking as a priority?

Help them to find ways to feel in better control of the situation. Critical thinking techniques can help them do that. For example, help them begin the shift with a plan—a clear plan for their priorities on that shift.

To assuage their frustration, tell them to elicit some of those priorities from patients. If they find out what is the one thing most important to each of the patients during the shift, they can be sure to address that short list and leave with the sense of satisfaction that comes from knowing they have met patient needs. This approach taps the critical thinking skill of considering multiple perspectives and there may be other relevant perspectives to seek on a given shift.

Another important part of the plan is identifying the absolute essentials of care to be performed. Sometimes nurses are tired before they start because they let *everything* be essential and important. New graduates particularly are plagued with this problem. This calls upon the critical thinking skill of analyzing. The approach also requires the critical thinking behavior of assembling evidence to support conclusions—that is, conclusions that you can defer certain routine matters. Making that judgment requires the courage of your convictions—another hallmark of critical thinking.

A third important part of the plan is identifying what tasks another can perform or if additional staffing is needed, what exactly is the need? For example, the need is *not* for one more LPN or one more RN—the need is for one-on-one care for a critically ill patient, or for Q 15 minutes vital signs on three patients. In other words, identify what specific assistance is needed. That makes it much easier for a staffing coordinator to assist the unit. There are usually plenty of alternatives to "X" number of additional RNs, LPNs, or UAP.

RESOURCES

Boucher, M. A. (1998). Delegation alert! *American Journal of Nursing, 98*(2), 30.

Carville, J., & Begala, P. (2002). *Buck up, suck up and come back when you foul up.* New York: Simon & Schuster.

Case, B. (1998). Competence development: Critical thinking, clinical judgment and technical ability. In K. J. Kelly Thomas, *Clinical and nursing staff development: Current competence, future focus* (pp. 240–281). Philadelphia: Lippincott.

Case, B. (2000). *Critical thinking: Working effectively with LPNs and UAP.* San Diego: Professional Development Center of American Mobile Healthcare (**www.rn.com**).

Covey, S. (1989). *The seven habits of highly effective people.* New York: Simon & Schuster.

Facione, P., & Facione, N. (1992). *The California Critical Thinking Disposition Inventory and CCTDI test manual.* Milbrae, CA: The California Academic Press.

Fisher, M. (1999). Do your nurses delegate effectively? *Nursing Management, 5,* 23–25.

Fonteyn, M. (1998). *Thinking strategies for nursing practice.* Philadelphia: Lippincott.

Haas, S., & Gold, C. (1997). Supervision of unlicensed assistive workers in ambulatory settings. *Nursing Economic$, 15*(1), 57–59.

Hansten, R., Jackson, M. (2004). *Clinical delegation: A handbook of professional practice* (3rd ed.). Sudbury, MA: Jones & Bartlett Publishers.

Helm, A. (1998). Liability, UAPs, and you. *Nursing, 11,* 52–53.

National Council of State Boards of Nursing. (1995). *Delegation: Concept and decision-making process, National Council position paper, 1995.* Chicago, IL: Author.

National Council of State Boards of Nursing. (1997). *Delegation decision-making grid.* Chicago, IL: Author.

Parsons, L. (1998). Delegation skills and nurse job satisfaction. *Nursing Economic$, 16*(1), 18–26.

Parsons, L. C. (1999). Building RN confidence for delegation decision-making skills in practice. *Journal for Nurses in Staff Development, 15*(6), 263–269.

Sheehan, J. (1998). Directing UAPs safely. *RN, 61*(6), 53.

Zimmerman, P. G. (1997). Delegating to unlicensed assistive personnel. *Nursing, 10*(5), 71.

Chapter 13: Selecting Practice Issues for Critical Thinking Application

"Pick battles big enough to matter, small enough to win."

—Jonathan Kozol, educator and award-winning nonfiction author

1. I think we definitely learn from our experiences with patients. It seems like we learn specific nursing techniques that work, certain monitoring with specific medications and other interventions. Isn't that a critical thinking process?

That is definitely a critical thinking process—one to celebrate and carry forward into ongoing practice. It is very important to identify and reflect out loud on critical thinking when it occurs. That helps make it visible, helps value it, and increases the likelihood that it will continue.

Go beyond highlighting the particular techniques you have found effective. Also highlight the process, the trial and error, the particular pieces of information nurses observed, and the outcomes obtained. Offer that model as one to use regularly as a means to improving care.

2. If I ask nurses how to improve care, they tell me they need more money and more help. How can I get them to focus on improvements in patient care?

You have to start where they are. Guide them in applying critical thinking strategies to the issues they've identified. In what specific ways will care improve if the nurses receive more money? On what basis can they justify more money? Local competitors? Professional organizations' data? The National Sample Survey? How does the benefit package fit into the picture? How do differentials for on-call, overtime, or other differentials compare with local, national, and specialty standards? How can they gain an audience with Administration and Human Resources to present their findings?

In what specific ways do they need more help? Is there any more effective way to use staff resources through assignments, delegation or selected use of personnel on duty in other capacities (such as the clinical nurse specialist or IV team)? In what specific ways will care improve if the nurse has more help?

If they had to choose more money OR more help which would they choose?

After you acknowledge and help them identify action steps to make the "more-money-more-help" mantra more than a gripe, ask for their specific suggestions to address the particular care improvements that you think are needed.

Focus on one needed improvement at a time and act on the suggestions you receive. This challenges your critical thinking. Restrain yourself from negating their suggestions with "We've never done it that way," or "That will never fly with the boss," or "We tried that once and it didn't work."

When nurses see you considering their suggestions and including them into new approaches, you will be reinforcing their efforts to think critically about improvements in care.

3. **Most of the nurses seem to think that the most important practice issues relate to new technology, treatments or diagnoses that are new to the unit. But, I'm not sure that we're doing the best we can with typical patients who are receiving familiar medications and treatments. How can I get the nurses interested in improving care for typical patients?**

Make a commitment to help the nurses add to their knowledge bases. Consult online resources in addition to professional journals. Share nursing implications of new findings, new techniques, and benchmark information in nurse-friendly forms: staff meeting announcements, posters, and short educational sessions in which you apply the new techniques and information to the care of a particular current patient.

Use an inquiring attitude in one-on-one exchanges with nurses and group meetings:

- Encourage the nurses to compare and contrast responses of different patients to the usual treatment regime. What accounts for the differences?
- Revise the usual practices in place for most typical patients. Are changes in practice indicated because of changes in circumstances, systems, length of stay, or other variables?
- What problems do the nurses, patients, patients' families, or any other parties experience with present practices in caring for typical patients? If you are not aware of perceptions of patients, families, and others involved in the care of typical patients, extend your inquiry to them. Encourage creative critical thinking to identify new approaches to these perplexing problems.

4. How can I get the nurses to apply their critical thinking skills to some quality improvement (QI) issues? They tell me they're too busy taking care of the patients and QI is for managers and administrators.

It's true that managers, administrators, quality improvement committee members, and others who work with QI projects and processes view the term in a different way than nursing staff do. People who are directly involved in the organization's QI processes take a more objective, proactive view.

Nurses sometimes view QI as critical of their efforts. Some nurses believe that they are giving absolutely the best care they can *under the circumstances* and perceive the message as "the quality of care you're delivering isn't good enough." So one way to ignite their interest in QI (after suspending use of the term) is to work with them to identify and set up indicators to take a look at some of those *circumstances*. In other words, what changes in the way we do things will improve patient care? What changes would empower nurses to give what they perceive as ideal, outstanding nursing care?

Obviously if there is need for improvement in compliance with safe practices or essential standards of care, the nurses *do* need to improve their practice. And I'm not suggesting sugarcoating that message. But, even if the nurses need to improve their practice, the quality improvement process is more than delivering that message. It includes looking for the causes of deviance from standards, collecting and analyzing data, trying some new approaches, and documenting and communicating the results.

After the nurses can see benefits to patients and to themselves, they will be more receptive to the QI label.

5. Lack of staff and lack of supplies seem to be pretty important practice issues on this unit. Can critical thinking approaches help solve those problems?

Definitely! Some might say that the critical thinking challenge is to create and improvise with what staff and supplies you have, and to some extent that may be a necessity. But the real critical thinking challenge is to identify the factors that contribute to the lack of staff and supplies and attack those problems.

Too often nurses work around the barriers. For example, if a nurse finds that he/she is wasting a lot of time at the automatic medication station or waiting for access to it, that nurse may decide to make only one trip per shift and fill pockets with all of the medications needed for that shift. You can probably think of many examples of nurses getting the job done in spite of the system. And while these efforts may permit the individual nurse to complete the shift assignment, these efforts do not get the problem fixed. Instead, these efforts perpetuate a broken system that requires constant effort to get the job done despite the broken system. That constant effort to maintain status quo can lead to burnout and a sense of hopelessness.

Critique the solutions to these problems that have been tried so far. Why have they not resolved the problem? What other information is needed? Who has the power to fix the problem? When it comes to the power to fix the problem, remember that power differs from authority. A coalition of staff members or a coalition of interdisciplinary colleagues may have the power to influence the formal authority to take actions to facilitate a solution. However, they can wield this power only with well-reasoned and supported recommendations.

6. Some days I barely find time to make rounds. How can I realistically fit critical thinking into my routine?

Use critical thinking to create your routine. Take a look at some of the suggestions in this chapter on setting priorities. You're certainly on the right track recognizing that rounds needs to be high on the priority list.

Rounds are definitely not expendable—though some frustrated managers and leaders let rounds take a back seat to attending meetings, working on the budget, interviewing applicants, filling staffing shortages, and other imperatives.

Plan rounds so that you gain the most information and make the most impact with the least expenditure of time. Make goal-oriented rounds. In the course of rounds, you'll collect information and advise staff on matters not directly related to the day's goal, but keep that focus. Knowing and acting on the clinical status of patients and their needs is really the core knowledge and action that propels you into interdisciplinary collaboration and empowers you to define staffing and budgetary needs. Rounds are also your opportunity to connect with staff at the heart of their work.

Let rounds be the organizer for your routine rather than the item you hope you'll find time for.

7. **I hate to admit it, but maybe I'm not as supportive of critical thinking as I could be. I guess the nurses are showing critical thinking when they circumvent the system to solve their own problems, but it doesn't help improve the system and sometimes their solutions increase the risk of mistakes. How can I encourage critical thinking and still maintain compliance with policies?**

You're on the right track here in recognizing that nurses are doing some critical thinking. But it sounds like their solutions are falling short of meeting a couple of important criteria: patient safety and compliance with policy.

You really cannot tolerate deviations from policy that create safety risks. One of the ways in which we protect safety is to standardize practices. It sounds like you may need to apply critical thinking skills to make changes in systems and policies.

It is not realistic to expect staff nurses to draft policies, but they have valuable input to offer about the problems they have experienced with present practices.

Ensure that the nurses understand that compliance with policy protects not only patient safety, but also protects them from legal risk. Make a commitment to the nurses that you will use their input to achieve systems changes and policy changes that protect safe practice and allow them to get their work accomplished.

In the meantime, can you standardize and pilot test some alternative practices to alleviate the problems?

8. **Is every practice issue a critical thinking issue? It seems to me that lots of practice issues arise because we don't follow our own policies and procedures.**

Every practice issue is not necessarily a critical thinking issue—but more issues may be amenable to critical thinking than we might think at first. High-risk, emergency situations require rapid decisive action. The protocols that govern those situations result from previous critical thinking processes and recognizing the cues that call for the protocol requires critical thinking. However, when the protocol goes into effect, one team member assumes leadership and others follow the direction rather than collaborate about what to do next.

Use critical thinking skills to tackle the issue you raise about failing to follow policies and procedures. Examine the reasons for lack of compliance with policy. Perhaps you need to make changes in systems, assignments or other changes to facilitate compliance. Or, perhaps you need to change policy.

9. Some of the nurses have the attitude, "Why should I go out on a limb questioning orders and policies—seems like I'm just asking for trouble!" How can I help them see the value in questioning?

Assure that there *is* value in questioning—value that they can see and appreciate. When questioning behavior is expected and rewarded, the value becomes evident and nurses enjoy the satisfaction of practicing their full professional roles. Ensure that they get the feedback that their questions lead to changes and make a positive difference in patient care.

Encourage them to question not only physicians, pharmacists, and members of other disciplines. Encourage them also to challenge nursing policies, practices, staffing, assignments, scheduling, and all of the other aspects of practice. To encourage that kind of behavior requires courage and true commitment to critical thinking. It requires open-mindedness and willingness to withhold the sometimes knee-jerk response of defending the way you're doing things, but it is essential to foster a critical thinking environment.

10. Isn't critical thinking mainly for root cause analysis and examining mistakes?

Critical thinking becomes highly visible in root cause analysis and in the process of examining mistakes because it is spelled out as an analytical, stepwise process. But, as you are finding in the many examples and recommendations in this book, critical thinking approaches can enhance patient care and nursing practice in many ways. Apply some of the steps in formal root cause analysis to tackle practice issues—for example, asking "Why?" until you get to the root of the problem.

However, resist the temptation to think of critical thinking as a prescribed, stepwise process. The various challenges that arise in practice call for different critical thinking behaviors at different times. For example, sometimes asking "What's wrong with this picture?" to identify risk or need for improvement; sometimes taking multiple perspectives to reach an effective solution; sometimes assembling evidence to support conclusions—all are critical thinking activities.

11. The biggest practice issues are systems problems and problems with other departments. How can working with the nurses on critical thinking help us?

It sounds as if the nurses have already been exercising the critical thinking skill of assembling evidence to support conclusions: the conclusion that the biggest practice issues are systems problems and problems with other departments. Beware of destructive finger pointing or gleeful tallying every time another department fails to deliver. Such attitudes and activities build defensiveness and interfere with interdisciplinary problem solving.

Ask the nurses what systems, procedures, options in the information technology system, or other improvements would solve what you are identifying as the biggest practice issues. Clarify the outcomes you will obtain with improved systems and interdepartmental interface. Then you will have a means of measuring the effectiveness of solutions that you try.

Ask the nurses also to identify what changes in practices or procedures nursing might make to work more smoothly with systems or with other departments. This is not the same thing as devising clever ways to get around system problems.

When you are clear on the desired outcomes, identify who else needs to be involved and who will represent the unit—the representative need not always be the manager.

Ensure that the nurses see the results of their input into identifying the problem and proposing solutions. Carry their input forward into the interdisciplinary problem solving arena. Give the nurses feedback on progress. Most systems and interdisciplinary solutions take time. Prevent the discouragement that can cause nurses to give up on critical thinking by keeping them advised of progress and projected timetables for implementing solutions.

When the organization is testing solutions to these problems, again the nurses are called upon to think critically—to critique the solutions. How well do they satisfy the criteria for an effective solution? How well are they achieving the desired outcomes?

12. Many of the nurses say they're too stressed out to think about new approaches to patient care. Can critical thinking strategies help alleviate stress?

Critical thinking strategies can indeed help alleviate stress. Assist the nurses to:

- Build and reflect on their knowledge base related to stress. Much new information has become available in recent years—particularly information about middle-aged women and stress. Since approximately 95% of the nursing workforce is female and the average age of nurses is in the mid-40s, this new information is relevant to nurses and those who manage them.

- Analyze work life and personal life for stressors. Build self-awareness of stress indicators and triggers. Make and act on some decisions about making some changes to eliminate stressors or manage them more effectively.

- Detach from the emotional response to stressful situations. Identify your role in the situation and set limits.

- Maintain an open-minded attitude toward stress management techniques. Some nurses are skeptical that techniques such as meditation, deep breathing and other relaxation techniques have value. There is a tremendous array of stress-relief measures. And, one size does not fit all—one technique may work impressively for one person and have no value for another. However, some techniques such as social support, finding outlets for stress, and gaining a sense of control seem to provide relief to most people. Part of gaining a sense of control can be achieved through the critical thinking technique of reframing the situation—looking for the positive aspects and modifying the situation to magnify those aspects.

- Reflect on the results they obtain using stress management techniques. If meditation does not seem to help, has the nurse given it a fair trial? It takes time to learn to meditate and make meditating a habit. Make a conscious effort to evaluate your response to various techniques—including measures taken to modify stressors.

- Practice self-care and positive health practices—including diet, exercise, and avoidance of excessive use of alcohol and other drugs.

13. The nurses say that the physicians make all the decisions anyhow so why bother with critical thinking when their thoughts don't affect the way the patients are managed?

No question that the final decision-making authority rests with the physician or other provider. *However*, nurses' input into those decisions is critical and often makes a significant difference in patient outcomes.

As a leader, model the behavior of questioning providers when you identify safety issues, significant assessment information, or other factors that belong in the decision-making process. Enforce the expectation that nurses ask questions.

Help the nurses build their skills in communicating with providers. This is not simply a matter of communication techniques. This is a matter of critical analysis of the situation. And then, articulate presentation of the relevant facts and *how these facts create a question in the nurse's mind.* This requires solid knowledge, assessment information, and courage. However, the rewards lie in improved patient outcomes, increased respect from providers, and enhanced professional self-esteem, not to mention the avoidance of negative consequences such as patient injury or death, incident reports, disciplinary actions, and malpractice claims.

14. The physicians have been complaining lately that the nurses don't have complete information when they call to report problems or findings. How can I help nurses think things through before they call the physicians?

Pin the physicians down to specifics. Don't get defensive; just find out what kind of information is lacking so that you can address the problem.

There are probably at least three components to the problem.

1. It may be that some of the nurses do not recognize pieces of information that are significant given the patient's condition.

2. It may be that some of the nurses know what information is significant but either do not know how or do not have time to obtain the information.

3. It may be that some of the nurses lack confidence and assertiveness when reporting to the physicians.

15. How do I get the physicians to help instead of just complaining?

Go beyond asking the physicians what information is lacking. Ask some questions about what kind of reports are most helpful to them. On an individual basis, physicians also may prefer different types of communication. Some prefer to be re-oriented to the patient's status (e.g., post-op day, what the resident did on rounds, or other reminders) rather than given a cryptic snapshot of a lab value or a blood pressure. You are creating a "communication preferences" list—a version of the surgeon's preferences lists used in the OR.

Communicate to the physicians that you will work with the nurses to improve reporting. And, communicate to them that since communication is a two-way process, you expect certain professional behaviors of them: courtesy as a baseline expectation, but also brief explanations of the importance of certain information that the nurse may have neglected to offer.

There is probably an educational component to this situation. You will determine how to educate the nurses based on your judgment. Depending upon the situation, approaches might include:

- Invite an MD or two to give a 10-minute inservice class in a staff meeting about "Monitoring and Reporting Findings on the Patient who has . . ."
- Role play rehearsals in the educational setting. Let the nurses role play real MDs. They will probably enjoy taking on the characteristics of their physician colleagues. Let the nurse in the MD role critique the report offered by another nurse.
- Identify the "stars"—that is, the nurses who give outstanding reports to physicians. Let them lead discussions that identify patient situations, the MD involved, and how to report. Place the stars in the role of critiquing "reports" constructed by pairs of nurses.
- Offer one of the numerous assertiveness training programs available. Seek recommendations from the staff development specialist or clinical nurse specialist.

16. I've read that case studies are good for teaching critical thinking. Isn't that too much of an academic approach for practicing staff nurses?

It's too much of an academic approach if you take the cases out of a book or source of case material other than the nurses' practice. Whoever is planning educational activities—the Nurse Manager, the Clinical Nurse Specialist, the Staff Development Specialist—needs to select case situations from the practice setting.

Certainly there is at least one patient per week on most units who presents opportunities for nurses to refine their critical thinking and clinical judgment skills.

Since you are probably restricted by short time frames for education and case discussions, focus on the aspect of the patient's situation that offers the best opportunities for analyzing and practicing critical thinking and clinical judgment. This does not usually require the full patient history. Rather than providing a large bolus of information, let the nurses ask for what else they think they need to know to make a judgment about the question you are raising. Identifying what else they need to know is a critical thinking activity.

Perhaps you cannot identify a real patient whose situation illustrates all of the factors that you want the nurses to consider. Instead of looking for, or constructing an academic case, simply pose those additional factors as "What ifs?" For example, "What if the physician decides to put this patient with diabetes on a beta-blocker?"

17. I need a manageable way to work with the nurses on critical thinking and clinical judgment. Can you recommend a sound bite, on-the-fly way to work on critical thinking and clinical judgment?

When we think about providing education for nurses, we seem to think first of classes and self-study programs. Today, staffing constraints make it difficult to provide those to nurses. And yet, even if classes and self-studies were viable options, I'm not so sure that they'd be more effective than purposeful bedside, "chart-side," or other one-on-one encounters with nurses on the unit, such as encounters with pairs of staff working together, a few nurses in the break room or medication room, or the group assembled for a staff meeting.

But it takes both commitment and a sound clinical knowledge base on the part of the leader, manager or educator to seize and use these opportunities to build critical thinking skills. Most practicing nurses learn better when they are learning instantly useful information relevant to the care of a patient.

The leader, manager, or educator who rises to this challenge needs to be armed with questions. But use those questions judiciously. Perhaps only one question at each encounter; for example:

- What else could be causing . . .?
- How will you evaluate this plan, response to this medication?
- What do you infer from the lab results this morning?
- How is this new ACE inhibitor different from the earlier generations?
- What herbs does this patient use? St. John's Wort can render this drug ineffective.
- What other perspectives do you need to consider?
- What is this patient's priority today?
- Or, construct a question related to the most essential aspect of care for that patient that day.
- Or, raise questions about alternate approaches to assignments, scheduling, or delegation.

Prepare the nurses for this approach. Otherwise they may perceive the questions as criticism of their practice and respond defensively. Nurses have experience in learning by the questioning method. It was probably a mainstay of the clinical instruction they received in nursing school. That fact may or may not increase their openness to the technique. Evaluate the effectiveness of the technique periodically. You will probably find that, for many staff, your questions have stimulated questions that they ask themselves and each other. And, if that is the result, you will have succeeded in fostering critical thinking.

18. We seem to have a hard time dealing with family members visiting. How can I encourage them to think differently about visitors?

Thinking differently about visitors requires that the nurses *think like* visitors. In other words, apply the critical thinking skill of taking multiple perspectives. There is no question that it is easier for the nurses to give care on their own schedules and without visitors interrupting care and questioning them.

And so when you raise the issue in a staff meeting, ask them to assume the visitor role for a few minutes. Ask them to imagine a significant other, relative or close friend as a patient in a critical care unit at another facility. Encourage them to do their best to set aside their nursing perspective and think like a visitor. Would they be able to arrange work schedule, transportation, and other responsibilities around the visiting hour schedule (assuming that the rules were the same as your unit uses)? What are their biggest concerns as visitors?

Then, let them go back to the nurse role. Use one of the models described in the chapter on critical thinking models to examine perspectives about visiting hours. The staff group might examine each perspective together, or you might direct nurses as individuals, in pairs, or groups of three to list all the relevant points from a single perspective—assigning each perspective to a different nurse, pair, or group of three.

After examining each perspective, consider how they fit together. Are there creative approaches to managing visiting hours that could accentuate the positives and minimize the negatives? What kind of visiting policies respect the feelings of all involved and still reflect the relevant facts and evidence about visitors and patient care?

Make the investment of time you spend examining the issue worthwhile. Identify a new approach or two to try out. It may not necessarily be a new schedule or new rules for visiting hours. It may be a new way of interacting with visitors while maintaining present visiting hours. Establish criteria and a time frame for evaluating the results of the trial.

19. I see some questionable judgment in some nurses' documentation. They seem to be so concerned about defensive documentation that their charting is more about what they did and how the system failed than the patient's condition and response to treatment. Are those examples of errors in judgment?

Those are examples of distrust, frustration, and a feeling of threat. If it's all about one department, physician, or system, address the root problem as well as the documentation issue. The documentation in a way is a cry for help—a plea to fix this.

Explore the issues that are creating the problems nurses are documenting. In the meantime, intervene immediately to correct the documentation practices.

I'm usually reluctant to call a problem an education or training issue because I have yet to find an issue without a management component. And, there is a management component here too—the manager must set and uphold documentation standards. The manager must periodically review documentation to ensure ongoing compliance, and identify and act on all opportunities to improve.

20. What about guidelines for documentation? Is that too prescriptive?

Staff need to learn clear documentation guidelines. The patient's medical record is about the *patient*. Nurses need to use the patient's medical record to document the patient's condition, treatment, and response to treatment. But nurses also need to know and use the proper mechanism for documenting near miss, chain-of-command, and other risk and quality improvement issues. They need to understand the difference, the reasons for the difference, and to act on those understandings.

This usually requires more than a presentation about what information goes where. Nurses need reassurance that keeping systems and staff competence issues out of the patient's record is not strictly a cover-up to reduce the organization's exposure to legal risk.

And, back to the management component—nurses need to see that improvements result when they use the proper channels for reporting issues.

21. Are there some general critical thinking strategies that nurses can use to improve their judgment with medication administration?

The major critical thinking strategy that will help is questioning—the attitude of inquiry that drives critical thinking. As basic as the Five Rights are, failure to observe them is often the root cause of errors. Some have proposed two additional rights: right indication and right documentation. No matter how basic it may appear, safety requires that nurses commit to asking themselves:

- Is this the patient for whom this drug is ordered?
- Is this the drug that is ordered? Similar sounding drug names, confusion about trade names and generic names, and illegible handwriting contribute to many errors.
- Is this the time for which this drug is ordered?
- Is this the dose that is ordered? If I calculated a dose or volume, did I or another nurse double-check my calculation? Some drugs have a very wide range of therapeutic dose; for others the range is very narrow. Some drugs are used in different dosages to treat different conditions. In a hurry, or when distracted, a nurse may inaccurately assume that the usual dose is the dose that was ordered.
- Is this the route that is ordered?
- What is the specific indication for this drug in this dose for this patient?
- Have I documented completely, including patient's response? Some nurses have followed the dangerous practice of documenting medications as given in advance of actually administering them.

The question, "What is the specific indication for this drug in this dose for this patient?" is one that some nurses think goes beyond the scope of their practice. They think that this is a question that belongs to the prescriber or the pharmacist. But the more complete form of that question is squarely within the province of safe nursing practice: "Should I question the prescriber or pharmacist about this order because there is no documented indication for this patient to receive this drug, or because the dose is unusual, or because I know information about the patient such as other drugs he/she is receiving or body system compromises (such as liver or renal disease) that create a risk in administering this drug to this patient?"

The nurse uses critical thinking skills to identify the need to question the order, and also to frame the question to the prescriber or pharmacist. To raise the question in a competent, professional manner the nurse assembles the evidence that supports the reasoning behind the question and the nurse persists in questioning the prescriber or pharmacist until the nurse is comfortable with the answer.

Another inescapable fact is that critical thinking operates on a knowledge base and uses facts and principles. Two questions are essential to safe practice: "What else do I need to know?" and "Where can I find that information?" There is no acceptable excuse for denying nurses access to up-to-date drug information. Whether on intranet, regularly updated reference books, online references, or clinical pharmacist or package inserts, nurses cannot practice safely without access to credible drug information. Some hospitals have improved medication safety by providing nurses with access to a unit-based clinical pharmacist.

RESOURCES

Case, B. (1995). Critical thinking: Challenging assumptions and imagining alternatives. *Dimensions in Critical Care Nursing, 14*(5), 274–279.

Case, B. (1999). *Preceptor workbook: Advanced practice nurse.* Chicago, IL: Loyola University of Chicago Marcella Niehoff School of Nursing.

Case, B. (2001). *Critical thinking: Managing stress.* San Diego: Professional Development Center of American Mobile Healthcare (**www.rn.com**).

Joint Commission on Accreditation of Healthcare Organizations. (2000). *Root cause analysis in health care: Tools and techniques.* Oakbrook, IL: Author.

Paul, R. (1995). *Critical thinking: How to prepare students for a rapidly changing world.* Santa Rosa, CA: Foundation for Critical Thinking.

Chapter 14: Collaborating for Effective Resolution

> *"The man who gets the most satisfactory results is not always the man with the most brilliant single mind, but rather the man who can best coordinate the brains and talents of his associates."*
>
> —W. Alton Jones, former president of Cities Services, parent company of Citgo gasoline stations, and outdoors enthusiast

1. What does collaboration really mean?

Figure 14-1 represents collaboration. Let the circle represent one of two parties who need to reach a mutually acceptable decision. The square represents another party. For the sake of simplicity, the diagram includes only two parties, but any number might be involved.

In order to collaborate, each party must identify the most important features of a solution that will be acceptable from his/her point of view. Suppose that you, as a staff nurse, are collaborating with a peer about the duties of a UAP who is working with both of you. Suppose that you each have initially identified that you need essentially a full shift's worth of time from the UAP. Each of you will have to think outside-the-box to resolve this. You each began with the usual duties of the UAP in the care of each patient assignment. But—the result is an untenable assignment for the UAP.

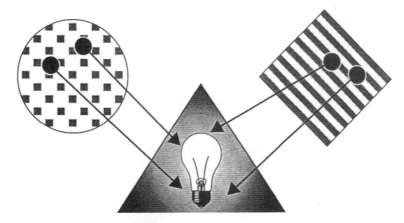

Figure 14-1: Collaboration

Let the diagram represent you as the circle and the other nurse as the square. The circles inside those shapes represent the most important specific features of a solution that each of you finds acceptable. The triangle represents the "table" upon which you each place those specifications. The light bulb represents the new ideas that you generate together—ideas that will satisfy the most important criteria for each of you.

To collaborate toward a solution, you must each identify what is most important in the situation. Take a step back from what it is you each intended that the UAP needed to do with patients. Instead focus on what is most important from each of your perspectives. What are the most important aspects of care for each of the patients? What are the essential RN functions? What lies within the UAP competency? What other constraints exist (e.g., schedules, your physical limitations, the other nurses, or the UAP)?

When each of you has identified the most important criteria, use those criteria as the specifications for a solution. The solution may involve each RN doing some usual UAP duties, or it may involve getting some more UAP assistance, or it may involve you and the other RN doing certain activities with one another's patients.

This is different from compromising. In compromising, each party simply gives up something. In collaborating, a new solution is achieved based on first identifying the most important ingredients of a solution for all parties involved.

2. Can't you truly collaborate only when the players have equal power?

Certainly equal power facilitates the spirit of collaboration, but it is not essential. At the very least the players share the goal of safe, effective, legal, high quality patient care. Sometimes reminding yourself and the other player or players of that common goal invites collaboration.

What is essential for collaboration is that the parties are stakeholders in the situation and that each one affects or is affected by the outcome.

3. How can you elicit collaborative behavior?

Invite the other party or parties to identify what is most important. Lead the collaboration process by offering an example—identify what is most important from your perspective. This does not mean simply justifying the solution you have initially proposed. It means taking a step back from *how* you want to accomplish your objective and identifying clearly *what* it is that you want to accomplish. There are probably several possible *hows* to achieve the *whats* that are most important to the parties involved.

4. Can you resolve most conflicts with a collaborative approach?

Not necessarily. Some urgent, high-risk situations call for decisive action by the best-prepared individual on the scene. Some disputes or conflicts are simply not important enough to warrant such investment of time and effort. Some issues are more important to one party than the other. Sometimes it makes sense to accommodate the preferences of another in order to store up good will for later use.

But on issues important to all parties concerned, the best way to an enduring solution is to collaborate. Lack of collaboration is sometimes the reason that problems keep "coming unsolved" or recurring.

5. I know that collaboration is a recommended style for conflict management, but I've also read that at least some research shows that nurses choose other styles more frequently. Why is that?

One study of nurses' most frequent conflict management styles (Fowler, Bushardt, & Jones, 1998) found that nurses most frequently resolved conflicts by avoiding, compromising, or accommodating. These are three of the five conflict management styles identified by Thomas and Kilmann.

The Thomas and Kilmann model of conflict management identifies five conflict management styles, each of which is a blend of two dimensions as shown in Table 14.1.

The styles that require a high degree of assertiveness were not the styles preferred by the nurses in the study.

TABLE 14.1   Conflict Management Styles

Conflict Management Style	Assertiveness:	Cooperativeness:
	The extent to which you identify and express your needs in the situation	The extent to which it is important to you to maintain a positive relationship with the other party
	(High, Medium, Low)	(High, Medium, Low)
Compromising	Medium	Medium
Accommodating	Low	High
Avoiding	Low	Low
Competing	High	Low
Collaborating	High	High

There are probably many reasons why many nurses experience difficulty in identifying and expressing their needs such as historical factors, gender-related typical behavior, physician dominance, altruistic motives, and other reasons.

Regardless of why a nurse might tend not to identify and express professional needs, collaboration *requires* that behavior and requires that the nurse develop skill in eliciting professional needs of members of other disciplines and of patients and their families.

6. Aren't all interdisciplinary efforts supposed to be collaborative?

Not necessarily. Please review my response to question 4. Some situations are more expediently, and just as satisfactorily, handled by compromising, accommodating, or accepting the direction of another party. However, for important, enduring decisions that require ongoing mutual cooperation, collaboration is the best choice.

And even when a less time-consuming strategy than full-blown collaboration is used, the *spirit* of collaboration adds to professional interdisciplinary decision making and planning.

As a party to interdisciplinary meetings, committees, and the like, empower yourself to participate and contribute actively. Too often nurses interpret their role as one of "representing nursing" or worse, being there only to "bring back information to nursing."

It *is* important to give the nursing perspective on the issues at hand and report the proceedings back to your nursing colleagues. But the spirit of collaboration requires more—it requires that you look at the problem with your interdisciplinary colleagues and enlarge your own perspective to view the situation from other perspectives. Palmer (1998) described this concept as viewing your own perspective as "a capacity to be enlarged [rather than] a scrap of turf to be defended" (p. 38).

7. Why can't we get the physicians to collaborate better with the nurses?

From surveying physicians on this issue one thing that I have learned is that physicians (and I suspect representatives of other disciplines as well) need some evidence of your competence before they are interested in collaborating with you. This means that professional rapport and mutual respect are preconditions for successful collaboration.

Someone has to initiate collaboration. Ask the physicians specifically what their needs are in particular patient management situations. Express the most important aspects from the nursing perspective.

The nurse manager's role is crucial both as a model of nurse-physician collaboration and as enforcer of the expectation that nurses and physicians collaborate.

8. Is it realistic to think that we really collaborate with UAP, technicians, and other unlicensed staff? Aren't they really here to follow directions?

Yes, they are here to accept appropriate delegation. But that does not erase needs that they may have in relation to their assignments. Their needs and your needs are the basis for collaborating. UAP may need feedback on specific aspects of their performance. They may need to feel a sense of control over certain aspects of unit routines. They may need direction about what to report to you regarding particular patients. They may need support and reinforcement in adapting to new duties or new ways of doing things.

Collaborating with UAP means finding out what their needs are in relation to working with you and expressing your needs in relation to working with them. And then, using both sets of needs as a framework, construct and agree to a plan for working together.

9. We seem to be expected to look outside our own walls more and more. We become part of one network, then another. What critical thinking approaches can help us collaborate with the constant change of players?

I think that my responses are beginning to sound like a broken record. The basis of collaboration is identifying and clarifying your own needs in the situation and then extracting from other stakeholders what it is that is most important to them in that situation. When the players are changing frequently, it becomes even more important to refine the skill of eliciting those needs and criteria from others and inviting them to collaborate toward a solution.

Also employ the critical thinking behavior of reflecting upon your needs and goals in light of the systems changes. Are the changes in affiliations changing your role or the scope of your responsibility? Perhaps these changes create some new or different needs and criteria from your perspective.

10. **It seems like every time we get a productive discussion going about how to improve care we get stymied by other departments' failures. I complain to other department managers and they just tell me why things are the way they are. Is there any realistic hope for collaboration in those situations?**

Hope lies in redefining the issues, rather than evoking the same old defensive responses. Complaints set up a defensive response. The customer service efforts directed toward handling complaints may have had some impact in responding to patient complaints or to criticism from supervisors, but it seems that peer-to-peer service complaints too often result in defensiveness, frustration, and little progress.

One worthwhile approach is to extend an olive branch of collaboration. Instead of complaining to the Radiology Department Manager about the long waits, ask, "What can we do to reduce the length of time that patients have to wait for X-rays? The patients get really uncomfortable and some are at risk for skin breakdown on those hard-surfaced carts. We're also running into problems with medications that need to be given on schedule. And some of these patients really need closer monitoring than we can accomplish when they are off the unit for such extended periods." In the question and statements, you are offering to help solve the problem and expressing why the delays create problems for you. You are also indicating what criteria are important to you in solving the problem: patient safety and comfort, timely medication administration, and monitoring.

Elicit a similar response from the Radiology Department Manager. What kinds of constraints and practices are creating the delays? Maybe other parties need to be involved in order to address the issue, such as the Patient Transportation Department or Information Technology if electronic scheduling is creating a problem.

Depending upon the constraints and causes, there are many possible solutions to this example issue. In some Radiology Departments, a nurse takes report and provides limited care for patients who need nursing care while in the Radiology Department. The parties involved need to evaluate all proposed solutions for their fit with the criteria that are most important to all parties.

Unfortunately, some managers are not receptive to peer invitations to collaborate. Persist for a while in attempting to elicit this new behavior. But, if a few tries yield no success, discuss the situation with your immediate supervisor. Perhaps the manager in question needs to hear from his/her boss that collaboration is an expectation.

11. I think we have some issues right here on the unit about working as a team. Can critical thinking approaches help us with that?

For teamwork to flourish, I think it has to be a management expectation. However, one researcher (Houser, 2000) found that teamwork and strong leadership from management were not related—at least in her study. But that finding perplexed the researcher and she intends to study that connection further. Perhaps a lack of strong leadership can force staff to work together. But in my experience, staff members usually give priority to the activities the manager values, expects, and rewards.

The manager needs to communicate not only the expectation, but also what that expectation looks like in practice. Consider:

- What are these issues you mention?
- Can you describe specifically what it would look like if those issues were resolved?
  - Would it be nurses asking one another if help is needed?
  - Or, nurses asking for help when they need it?
  - Or, a nurse who is uncertain about how to perform a particular procedure asking for support from a peer who has that particular expertise?
  - Or, more cooperation in creating the work schedule?

You will communicate much more effectively if you frame the expectation in specific behaviors rather than as the abstraction of "teamwork."

12. I know that determining goals and desired outcomes is a critical component for individual staff development. Does this fit with teamwork too?

Yes, you can also facilitate teamwork by helping staff members identify and agree to work toward a common goal or two—the more specific, the better. It is not realistic to think that all staff will perceive the same goals as important, but it is certainly possible to gain consensus and willingness to put forth effort on a limited number of goals. (See the technique suggested in question 6 of Chapter 12 on setting priorities.)

Some goals are really mandates—such as, reduce medication errors. It's best to acknowledge that fact. But, even though staff members had no say in identifying the goal, they can certainly offer valuable input to defining the various strategies that will help accomplish the goal. They can experience the satisfaction of working together in ways that they have suggested in service of a common goal.

13. **As a preceptor, I could sure use some collaborative help from my peers. I feel as if I'm left alone with the responsibility for orienting someone new. Sometimes the orientee and I even get a bigger assignment because there are two of us. How can the nurses who aren't precepting get involved?**

A functioning new staff member benefits all members of the staff, and all staff have a responsibility to invest in that new staff member. The manager needs to demonstrate some leadership in that regard—communicate and enforce the expectation that all staff have a role in bringing the new staff nurse up to speed.

The staff members who are not precepting can impart their special expertise—arrange for the orientee to accompany other staff members to watch expert performance of patient teaching, tricky IV starts, or other special skills. The orientee gains the opportunity to learn from expert performance and perhaps can plan to work on a particular skill with the other colleague. In addition, the orientee learns first-hand the special expertise of co-workers and, therefore, is learning to whom to call on for various kinds of assistance. Another staff member can also function as associate preceptor when the preceptor and orientee are not scheduled together. Orientation progresses smoothly and the orientee feels more comfortable when someone is designated to work with him/her in the preceptor's absence. To make most effective use of the associate preceptor, brief the preceptor on the orientee's progress and needs to date. Staff members can also facilitate precepting by taking on additional patient care duties to free the preceptor for precepting. All of these approaches require critical analysis of the orientee's needs and the resources of other staff members and then, collaborative planning based upon the needs identified.

14. **Benchmarking gets so much attention. Are there collaborative ways that we can approach benchmarking and performance improvement?**

When you compare the performance of the organization with benchmarks, you will likely discover that interdisciplinary collaboration has figured into the outstanding outcomes. Medication error reduction strategies provide a good example of outstanding outcomes produced through collaboration.

In some facilities, nurses' near-misses with look-alike drugs have led to packaging techniques in the Pharmacy Department to differentiate the drugs or to changes in vendors. Collaboration among administration, nursing unit management, Pharmacy Department, staff nurses, and clinical pharmacists has produced unit-based clinical pharmacist models that have significantly reduced medication errors in intensive care units. Collaboration among information technology (IT), medical records, laboratory, pharmacy, and nursing has led to forcing-function techniques that prevent errors.

When you compare your performance with benchmarks, use the critical thinking skill of analyzing. Determine *how* the outcomes in the benchmarks were achieved—for example, who collaborated with whom to get the job done? And, what milestones and intermediate goals were set and achieved on the way to success? Most of the indicators on which we compare ourselves with benchmarks have systems components. System fixes usually require collaboration.

Undoubtedly, your organization differs in at least a few ways from the benchmark. Here's where the creative part of critical thinking—looking at alternatives—becomes important. Although the organization differs from the benchmark, the intermediate goals that were set and achieved are still useful. You may need to employ some different approaches to achieving the milestones and intermediate goals. The process of collaborating with colleagues in other departments will lead to those alternate approaches.

15. How can I sort out what's truly relevant to my job so that I can collaborate with others more effectively?

It's easy to get distracted from your goals with the flood of information available today. The critical thinking skill of continually reflecting will assist you to keep your goals clearly in view.

What are your goals? Evaluate the flood of information in light of your goals. Also be alert for information that might indicate a need to reconsider your goals—new techniques, new populations, new services, and other new developments that affect the scope of your job.

With the capabilities of information technology, there is often much more information available than has any practical value. This is true of clinical information as well as information produced for management purposes. But this does not mean you can assume that new levels of detail have no value. Apply the critical thinking skill of questioning. Question the source of information—whether that source is the diagnostic radiology department, the materials management department, the staffing office, or the finance department. Ensure that you understand what the data represent and what significance they may have for you.

Don't be timid about seeking clarification—whether from the direct source of information or from a boss about expectations for the use of information.

Increase your skill in accessing information—on the Web as well as in the organization. When you feel confident in your ability to access the information you need when you need it, you won't feel as daunted by the constant onslaught of information or need to read, digest, and file everything that enters your visual field.

If you are in a management position and find it feasible to delegate, consider designating members of the staff to receive, review, and report to you on certain categories of information—for example, information technology (IT) or pain management.

16. We have increasing mandates to collaborate with patients and their families. Isn't this just advocacy?

Yes, advocacy—one of nursing's greatest strengths—is involved in collaborating with patients and their families. And perhaps your definition of advocacy includes the collaborative aspects. However, just let me emphasize those collaborative components.

Collaboration goes beyond helping patients and their families give voice to their preferences and needs. When you collaborate, you assist patients and their families to identify and articulate their most important needs in the situation. This sometimes takes ongoing exchange and clarification.

You also have a professional obligation to relate pertinent information to patients and their families that may modify their preferences and decisions. For example, suppose a post-op patient refuses a prescribed dose of ascorbic acid. She asks what that pill is. And, when you tell her ascorbic acid or vitamin C, she says, "I don't take that at home—I eat lots of citrus fruit and I don't want to take more vitamins." Rather than simply supporting her right to refuse, explain the rationale for the order—that ascorbic acid supports wound healing.

Don't mistake my suggestion as encouraging you to persuade patients and their families to accept care plans without question. What I'm suggesting is that we assist patients and their families to clarify their needs and give them the information they need to make fully-informed decisions.

17. I don't think patients and their families really want the responsibility of collaborating with us. They seem to want us to tell them what to do. Don't they really like it better when the nurses take charge?

There's no question that patients and their families want to believe that the nurses are competent and confident in providing care. There are certainly individual differences in deference to medical authorities related to personality and culture.

However, adverse publicity about healthcare has raised public concern and many patients feel at risk when they enter a hospital or healthcare environment. Some of this fear can be allayed by providing information on an ongoing basis, by asking for patient and family preferences, and by respecting those preferences whenever possible. It's really that same collaborative process that I've described repeatedly in this chapter: Find out what is most important to them, offer clarifying information as appropriate, and plan with them to meet the needs most important from your perspective and from theirs.

18. I think I could probably benefit from collaborating with my manager peers, but many of them seem so defensive and secretive about how they handle issues. How can I invite collaboration when some of my peers keep shutting down when I approach them?

Many managers find it difficult to acknowledge their own uncertainties with their peers. Unfortunately, there are those who prefer to maintain their own superiority by failing to help others grow in the management role. Certainly it helps if both the boss and the boss of your potential collaborative partner expect collaboration, support it, and set the stage for it.

Some of the approach, of course, depends upon individual personalities. Usually some version of "I'd just like to run this by you—you seem to handle situations like this one with ease. Here's what I think I'll do . . . What do you think?" works best.

It's always useful to state what you plan to do, or what you have tried without success. In this way, you are not asking a peer to solve your problem. Be sure to state clearly what it is you are trying to accomplish—your goals and needs in the situation about which you are seeking advice.

In approaching a seasoned manager, you might also describe an approach you read about or heard about at a conference. Ask the manager how he/she thinks that approach would be useful in the situation in question.

Don't forget that managers in other departments face many of the same trying situations that nurse managers face. They are useful potential collaborative partners as well. Building relationships around management issues makes a strong foundation for later collaboration on interdisciplinary issues.

19. **Some of the staff have the attitude "It's not my patient!" when they are asked for help or information related to patients who are assigned to other nurses. How can I create a better atmosphere for the staff to consider all the patients "our patients" on this unit and to take pride in the care of all patients even though another nurse is assigned to a particular patient?**

Expect and reward behaviors that express the sentiment that "these are our patients and we work as a team." Identify for staff the specific behaviors you hope to see. Resist the temptation to phrase the expectations as correction of interactions you have observed.

Instead develop "perfect world" scenarios of what mutual responsibility and teamwork look like. Describe this vision to the staff. Invite them to give you specific examples of what their vision of teamwork looks like. Ask them to tell you what the barriers are toward attaining that vision in practice. Ask what you can do as manager to contribute to achieving that vision.

Ask staff what advantages and disadvantages they perceive in practicing as a team. Reward every effort you observe toward improved teamwork and be sure to work hard at observing!

On the matter of rewards, do some inquiry and analysis with staff. Find out what they perceive as satisfying and rewarding. Rewards only do their job when the recipient perceives value in the reward.

20. **We're really feeling the effects of the nursing shortage. Can collaborative strategies offer any help?**

The nursing shortage certainly challenges us in many ways and provides opportunities for critical thinking. Both the right brain, creative aspects of critical thinking, and the left brain, logical aspects, come into play.

The logical aspects set parameters of patient safety, caregiver competencies, numbers of staff, numbers of patients, and perhaps other "givens" as well. The creative part is stepping outside of the usual ways of assigning patient care activities and complying with routines.

Times when staffing is less than optimal call for clear identification of priorities and collaborative plans for addressing priorities. Find out what is most important to each patient for this shift. Do all of the routine activities usually performed by UAP need to be done on this shift? Considering the patients' priorities and patient safety, are there more important ways to use UAP skills on this shift? Are there any resources available in the facility that you can tap—even for a limited period of time? For example, can you find a CNS to do a dressing change, a supervisor to give a medication, or a staff development instructor to monitor Q 15 minute vital signs?

Doing things differently requires collaboration of all parties concerned—identifying needs of each party and then buying into a plan that will meet the most important needs of all while acting within the criteria of patient safety and staff competencies. Collaborating with potential partners outside the walls offers many benefits. Consider community, professional organizations, nursing schools, and other potential partners.

21. **I can collaborate pretty well with my peers on my own unit, but when I get floated, I feel like the unit staff just close ranks and give me the assignments they don't want. Sometimes I don't even feel safe. How can I even begin to collaborate with nurses whom I don't know and won't be working with for the long term?**

First things first. If you don't feel safe do not let that feeling persist. Identify to the unit staff what your needs are and what contributions you can make to patient care. If you don't have all the specialty skills of the unit staff (and chances are you don't), then they may have to do some of the care for patients who are assigned to you. What can you do for patients they're assigned to in return? Are there other unit routine duties that are familiar that you could do for the unit staff to enable them to help you complete the care for patients assigned to you?

It's true that you won't be working with these nurses for the long term, but you all have to survive the shift—do better than merely survive. It's important to start off on the right foot. In the ideal world, they would welcome you. They would ask about your competencies and the specialty-specific skills that you may lack. They would give you appropriate assignments, tell you about priorities, and offer to help you. They would express their heartfelt gratitude for your work on their unit. And now back to reality! If you are not greeted in this way, what can you do to elicit that type of response from the nurses?

You can tell them about the things you wish they would ask you—your competencies, the specialty-specific skills you lack. You can ask them the things you wish they would tell you—priorities, help that you need, and so on. Granted you should be a welcome asset, but if it doesn't happen, rise above your disappointment. Model collaborative behavior for your hosts.

RESOURCES

Case, B. (2000). *Critical thinking: Mastering floating.* San Diego: Professional Development Center of American Mobile Healthcare (**www.rn.com**).

Case, B. (2000). *Critical thinking: Addressing staffing issues.* San Diego: Professional Development Center of American Mobile Healthcare (**www.rn.com**).

Case, B. (2000). *Critical thinking: Working effectively with LPNs and UAP.* San Diego: Professional Development Center of American Mobile Healthcare (**www.rn.com**).

Case, B. (2001). *Critical thinking: Managing stress.* San Diego: Professional Development Center of American Mobile Healthcare (**www.rn.com**).

Fowler, A. R., Bushardt, S. C., & Jones, M. A. (1998). Retaining nurses through conflict resolution. *Health Progress, 74*(5), 24–29.

Hansten, R., Jackson, M. (2004). *Clinical delegation: A handbook of professional practice* (3rd ed.). Sudbury, MA: Jones & Bartlett Publishers.

Houser, J. L. (2000). An evaluation of the relationship of the context of nursing care and patient outcomes. *Quest for Quality* sponsored by Mayo Continuing Nursing Education. November 4, 2001.

Leape, L., Kabcenell, A., Berwick, R., & Roessner, J. (1998). *Breakthrough series guide: Reducing adverse drug events.* Boston, MA: Institute for Healthcare Improvement.

Palmer, P. (1998). *The courage to teach.* San Francisco: Jossey-Bass.

Thomas, K., & Kilmann, R. (2002). *Thomas-Kilmann conflict mode instrument.* Toronto, Canada: Career/LifeSkills Resources, Inc.

Chapter 15: Evidence-Based Practice

"Truth will always be truth, regardless of lack of understanding, disbelief or ignorance."

—W. Clement Stone, 1902–, U.S. entrepreneur

1. Evidence-based practice has become quite a buzzword. What exactly does it mean?

I like the way the Evidence-Based Practice Medicine Group of McMaster University defined it (Hadwiger, 1999).

The Group identified that evidence-based practice involves:

"Collection, Validation and Interpretation

of

Valid, Important, Applicable Evidence

that is

Patient-reported, Clinician-observed or Research-reported" (p. 48).

Further, that evidence-based practice occurs when the "best available evidence, moderated by patient circumstances and preferences, is applied to improve the quality of clinical judgments and facilitate cost-effective care" (p. 48).

I like this definition because it honors evidence collected outside of formal research studies. It suggests that practitioners have a responsibility to perform their own practice not only with research findings, but also with their own systematic observations.

I don't mean to imply that clinicians' anecdotal observations equal the evidence produced in controlled, rigorous research. Certainly the main thrust of evidence-based practice is to incorporate research findings into practice. But I think it's important to consider the use and collection of evidence as an attitude toward practice—a way of practice that brings critical thinking to life.

I also like Ingersoll's (2000, p. 152) definition, "Evidence-based practice is the conscientious, explicit and judicious use of theory-derived, research-based information in making decisions about care delivery to individuals or groups of patients and in consideration of individual needs and preferences."

2. Isn't this evidence-based practice a fad that's likely to pass?

I hope not! Evidence-based practice is a hallmark of professional practice and high quality patient care. I hope that leaders in clinical facilities will embrace evidence-based practice and ensure that we are witnessing the beginning of a trend, rather than a passing fad.

Evidence-based practice shows respect for the practice of nursing. Evidence-based practice is a solid foundation for interdisciplinary collaboration. Evidence-based practice can help raise the professional profile of nursing practice and in so doing assist in attracting people to the profession who will ensure the continuance of the trend.

3. What's the difference between evidence-based practice and quality improvement?

Certainly the two are related. After identifying a problem or opportunity for improvement, the quality improvement process begins with measurement using relevant indicators in order to establish a baseline. After studying the contributors to the problem and introducing improvement, measurement is repeated in order to document improvement. As you can see, the process is very much like a research experiment. The difference is that no control groups, randomization or elaborate statistical procedures are usually included in the quality improvement process. Quality improvement takes place in the practice arena and it is usually not practical to control the many variables that affect outcomes.

The research process is more rigorous (see Chapter 16). Although quality improvement processes do include reviews of current literature, the reviews in research studies are much more extensive. Permissions from subjects are sought in research, but in quality improvement projects, the improvements that are introduced are more in the nature of a new way of doing things, such as an updated procedure or practice. Permissions that patients sign upon admission cover their consent to hospital policies.

Evidence-based practice and quality improvement share a focus on measurement and an insistence upon solid rationale for action.

4. Is evidence-based practice the same as gathering data to support an assessment or drawing conclusions about a patient's response to treatment?

Nurses who think critically make a practice of assessing patients thoroughly and evaluating patients' responses to treatment. Experienced nurses use a backlog of evidence they have collected and related to patient outcomes through their own direct observations.

The definition of the Evidence-Based Practice Medicine Group of McMaster University (Hadwiger, 1999) cited in response to question 1 embraces the concept of clinicians acting on evidence they have collected in their practice. But individual clinicians' observations are not a substitute for findings of controlled, large sample research studies that have some basis for external validity (i.e., for generalizing and applying findings and recommendations beyond the specific subjects studied).

I think that the optimal evidence-based practice environment uses relevant findings of reported research and encourages clinicians to interpret and incorporate the evidence they assemble when they examine their own practice. I think that application of published research findings needs to be complemented with an overall evidence-based approach to practice that includes alertness for evidence in one's own practice.

5. I attended a quality improvement meeting during which a couple of members got into a heated dispute about whether some findings were research or evaluation. What exactly is the difference?

Research generates new knowledge or validates previous research findings in new or expanded settings. Much of the research process takes place before data are actually collected. Evaluation makes a judgment about a project, program, or service that either has been completed or is in progress.

Evaluation takes place when the process, programs or outcomes to be evaluated have been in progress long enough to make evaluation meaningful. Criteria for evaluation are established and then evaluation is undertaken. The evaluation process usually includes observation of the program or service in operation.

Evaluation is more sound if it is planned before the outset of a program or service. Before the program begins, objectives for the program are stated and methods for measuring those objectives are identified. For example, Ulsenheimer and colleagues (1997) suggested some possible measurable outcomes for evaluating the impact of the introduction of a critical thinking model in the nursing department. But sometimes in the practice setting, programs or services change over time without careful consideration and planning of the evaluation process.

Research studies usually include more extensive literature reviews, larger samples, and a more rigorous control of variables. Some of the same distinctions I made in contrasting research and quality improvement also apply when differentiating research and evaluation.

The two are certainly closely related and, in fact, some projects are referred to as evaluation research.

6. How does evidence-based practice relate to critical thinking?

One of the characteristic behaviors of critical thinkers is the act of gathering evidence to support conclusions. Nurses use this behavior when they analyze assessment data and come to conclusions about patient response, patient problems, nursing diagnosis, and patient outcomes.

Evidence-based practice employs that skill and extends it to taking a perspective beyond the individual patient. That is, gathering evidence to support conclusions about (for example) the nursing care delivery model in use, the policy for monitoring patients who are receiving narcotics, or other specific nursing practices and products.

Critique is another important critical thinking behavior. In evidence-based practice, nurses make a habit of critiquing present practice and policy. They also critique research findings for their applicability to a particular patient population.

7. I always thought that intuition was an important part of nursing practice. Is evidence-based practice at odds with the concept of intuition?

In a word, no. I think that evidence-based practice challenges us to examine our intuition and attempt to make it explicit. One way to illustrate this is to refer to the model that describes the progression from unconscious incompetence to conscious unconscious competence (see Figure 15-1).

I think that intuition definitely has a hallowed place in expert practice. I also think that consistent with evidence-based practice we need to reflect on our intuition and articulate some of its components. Some of what we articulate might well be fodder for further research.

8. Surely you can't expect staff nurses to somehow find the time, energy, and resources to engage in research! How does this apply practically at the staff nurse level?

I agree that at this point in our history, staff nurses have neither time, energy, nor resources to engage in research. Even if they did, few are trained in research. And, in the present environment, it is unrealistic to expect that much education, training, or participation in the formal research process is feasible for staff nurses who have basic educational preparation.

Unconscious Incompetence

When you don't know what you don't know.

(e.g., your first day in ICU)

↓

Conscious Incompetence

You now know what information you don't know.

(e.g., your second day in ICU—now you're ready to learn, because you know what it is that you need to learn)

↓

Conscious Competence

Now you have learned some of the information you need to get started.

(e.g., as your orientation to ICU progresses and continues for a year or two—now you're ready to get started and move forward, but you must remain consciously aware of the information, mentally rehearse, and consciously think through. This is similar to Benner's (1989) competent level of practice in the novice-to-expert formulation.)

↓

Unconscious Competence

With experience, you now practice without consciously recognizing and reacting to cues. You identify patterns, often before concrete, explicit evidence presents itself.

(e.g., you consistently and intuitively recognize when a patient's condition is on the verge of deteriorating. You anticipate and address risk situations. This is similar to Benner's (1989) expert level of practice.)

↓

Conscious Unconscious Competence

By reflecting on your practice, you have identified and can articulate some ingredients of your intuition. You can describe and communicate to novices some of the subtle cues and patterns that comprise aspects of your intuition.

(e.g., you name the subtle signs and patterns you observe when a patient's condition is on the verge of deteriorating)

Figure 15-1: A View of Developing Competence. Note: From *The empathic communicator* (pp. 20–33), by W. S. Howell, 1982, Belmont, CA: Wadsworth Publication Company. Copyright 1982 by Wadsworth Publication Company. Adapted with permission.

But evidence-based practice is a way of practice, just as critical thinking is a way of practice. Nurse managers, CNSs, staff development specialists, and/or other leaders have the responsibility of assisting staff to integrate findings into practice and to align policies with research findings. The assistance to the nurses occurs most effectively at the bedside and not in an inservice class.

Staff nurses need to remain flexible and willing to embrace evidence-based changes in practice. They also need to take an evidence-based attitude toward their practice: to observe and report what works and what does not. The manager can facilitate this with periodic staff meeting agenda items such as "In what specific ways is the new IV pump better than the one we were using?"

Leadership that encourages this attitude is essential. When nurses see results based on their observations, they are motivated to continue an evidence-based attitude. For example, new products and pharmaceuticals often appear on the unit simply because the materials management department struck a great deal with the vendor. However, if the nurses document that the great new tape does not stick, or the packaging of IV drugs from the new vendor is creating near-misses because of look-alikes, and the manager forwards this information leading to changes, the nurses will experience their power in influencing patient care.

Leaders need to continually raise questions with staff. For example, "Why are some of the patients doing better than others after this type of surgery?" or "What did we do differently with Mrs. Hopkins this time to prevent her from falling?"

9. I'm in staff development and we always seem to be looking for evidence to support the effectiveness of educational programs. Any suggestions?

Bravo! You're looking for evidence. That's how staff development departments flourish—by documenting their effectiveness in terms meaningful to the organization, which is usually not head counts of attendance and positive evaluations about the learning experience.

Just as you plan learning experiences beginning with the objectives, you need to plan evidence gathering for effectiveness (also known as outcome and impact evaluation). Outcome evaluation answers the question, "Do they do it on the unit?" and impact evaluation answers the question, "So what?" given that the nurses accomplished the objectives of an educational session; that is, given that the participant and instructor evaluations of the learning activity were positive, and the post-test results were satisfactory, and the nurses are using what they have learned in their practice.

What impact is there upon organizational goals such as length of stay, nosoco-mial infection rate, medication errors, worker's compensation claims, and other organizational goals?

Planning evidence gathering in advance allows you to establish a baseline. Identify at least one valid, meaningful measure that will allow you to track the impact of educational programming.

Remember that staff development faces a double challenge when it comes to evidence-based practice. One part of the challenge is assisting staff to integrate research findings into practice—this may require leadership in initiating policy changes that reflect alignment with research findings. The second part is inte-grating findings related to educational approaches and the impact of education in staff development practice.

10. Evidence has such a courtroom-drama, litigious sound to me. Doesn't it seem related to gathering evidence against individual staff members in some sort of disciplinary process?

Unfortunately some of us practice in defensive environments. There is a certain "write 'em up" mentality that dominates some practice settings. Leaders are responsible for setting a more positive tone, beginning with more careful and selective hiring practices.

One of the main foci of the recent attention to medical errors has been the need to create a culture of safety in which we truly view mistakes as opportunities to improve. Even to establish meaningful baseline data about errors, clinicians must be willing to *report* errors and near-misses.

A culture that views errors as opportunities to improve presupposes that indi-viduals who practice in that culture are competent to perform their jobs and willing to do so. Leaders need to select, train, and support clinicians and assis-tive personnel for safe, high quality patient care. And, unfortunately, this approach may include disciplining, remediating, counseling, and possibly dis-missing staff members who are incompetent and unwilling to develop or demonstrate the competency that the job requires.

11. This idea of integrating research into practice seems idealistic to me. How can you make this more realistic and achievable?

Gennaro (1994) cited Hunt's (1981) research that identified five reasons why nurses do not use research findings in practice:

1. They do not know about them.
2. They do not understand them.
3. They do not believe them.
4. They do not know how to apply them.
5. They are not allowed to use them.

I think that all of these reasons create barriers. It is hoped that nursing education instills a responsibility for lifelong learning and the rudiments needed to critique and apply pertinent research findings. But realistically, the practice environment needs to assist and support nurses in their use of research in practice.

Nursing leaders need to commit to creating an evidence-based practice culture. This means employing the techniques suggested in this chapter.

Alfaro-LeFevre (2003) offered a useful tool in assisting nurses to critique research findings. The matter of setting the expectation and initiating a policy making process that responds to research findings rests with leadership.

12. Whose responsibility is it to integrate research into practice?

If I say it is everyone's responsibility, that would seem to make it no one's responsibility. But I do believe that nurse managers, CNSs, staff development specialists, staff nurses, and others have responsibilities within their own roles to identify and apply research findings and to foster an environment for evidence-based practice. It helps greatly to spell out the responsibilities of various roles.

For example, it may be the role of the manager to raise questions about products, policies, practices, or observations about differences in patient outcomes. The role of the CNS and/or staff development specialist may be to identify pertinent findings, communicate them to staff in a meaningful way, and follow up with bedside consultations. Any of these leaders may have the responsibility for bringing policies and procedures into alignment with research findings.

The role of the staff nurse is to raise questions, critique policies and practices, and develop the habit of evidence-based practice. Ideally, staff nurses read research in their specialty and determine:

- whether the findings apply to the patients (by comparing the patient population with the sample studied)
- whether they understand the findings and conclusions
- whether implementing the recommendations will improve the care they deliver

Then, they should ask for assistance from their leaders in interpreting and applying research findings. Leaders need to encourage nurses to read, critique, and apply research, but must recognize that setting unrealistic expectations for nurses will not accomplish the goal of integrating research into practice.

The specifics of role responsibilities vary with the setting, but in general the manager's role is to expect, enforce, and create an environment that supports evidence-based practice. The CNS's and/or staff development specialist's role is to supply nurses with ready-to-use research findings and to support the staff in inquiring and critiquing. The staff's role is to incorporate applicable research findings into practice and develop an evidence-based practice attitude. The CNS and/or staff development specialist may also have the responsibility of actually engaging in research or in developing pilot projects to evaluate various techniques and products.

13. It's great to say we should be integrating research into practice here, but we have policies and procedures to consider. Should we really be encouraging staff to apply research findings even if our policies differ from research recommendations?

I think you're really asking, "How do we integrate research findings when policies conflict with research recommendations?" Nurses must practice within the facility's policies and procedures in order to protect themselves and the facility from legal risk and from risk of noncompliance with accreditation standards. However, someone needs to take responsibility for keeping a watchful eye on research findings and drive policy changes accordingly. CNSs are probably the ideal candidates for the job, but all services in all facilities do not have designated CNSs.

Maybe the process for updating policies and procedures needs to be updated itself. The process should not present a barrier to integration of research findings.

I also encourage you to take a close look at the policies. Are they really so specific as to prohibit use of new findings? Sometimes routine "way we've always done it" practices become sacred, even though they are not dictated by policy. For example, research as long ago as 1983 and later replicated indicates that breastfeeding problems occur more frequently when mothers and babies are separated, when there are delays in initiating breastfeeding, and when the duration of breastfeeding is limited, yet these findings are not acted upon in all facilities nearly 20 years later (Gennaro, 1994). Is policy the only impediment?

14. What are some practical techniques for raising awareness of research findings?

It depends somewhat on the setting and also on where in the facility information catches the nurses' attention: the coffee room, the med room, the intranet, a bulletin board in the nurses' station, staff meeting announcements, a paycheck insert, or whatever locations have proven successful. For these vehicles, the message must be concise and directly applied. For example, a message in any of those locations that says, "Did you know that one facility decreased its use of Narcan to near-zero by instituting Q1H respiratory rate observations on all patients who receive narcotics?"

It works best to give one message at a time. Use succinct, attention-getting language. Depending upon the particular finding on which you are focusing, it might be the focus for a week, a month, or a quarter. In the case of the narcotics monitoring example above, a theme of narcotics safety could continue for a quarter—including many aspects such as generic/brand name confusion, sign-out procedures, MAR recording, pain management protocols (another area in which much research has been reported), and any other aspects of narcotic safety that have been troubling.

Also, build research findings into all inservice presentations—however brief. The aim is to *integrate* research findings and not to make research a separate topic.

Again, the most important method for imprinting the use of research findings and the spirit of evidence-based practice is working alongside staff, offering consultation and raising questions about practice.

15. Some CNSs used to facilitate journal club meetings in which the staff discussed research articles. What are some alternatives for sharing research?

CNSs, nurse managers, staff development specialists, and other nursing leaders need to empower and support nurses in making observations about the effectiveness of present practices and in integrating research findings into practice.

The most effective way to do this is to meet the nurses at the bedside with questions and with recommendations coming from research. Short segments of staff meetings, inservice sessions, intranet announcements, and posted bullet points can be vehicles for collecting observations and for communicating findings, but if evidenced-based practice is to become a habit, nurses need encouragement and reinforcement at the bedside in the care of patients.

16. Is it realistic for staff development specialists and CNSs to be conducting research? We do have statements to that effect in their job descriptions.

It really depends upon the preparation of those individuals, the setting, and the other requirements of their jobs. It seems to me that these roles are accountable for identifying and facilitating application of pertinent research findings. Some facilities have nurse researchers on staff. Certainly in those facilities, the nurse researcher can direct others in the research process and in applying research findings. There may be opportunities for Staff Development Specialists and CNSs to partner with other nurse researchers as a part of university-based research projects.

Job descriptions should reflect the possible and not the perfect world ideal. If the performance of those professionals is to be evaluated using the statements and criteria in the job description (and of course that should be the case), then the job description should clearly state the accountabilities and expectations. It only waters down the meaning of research to state in a job description that the incumbent in a position "engages in research," if such activity is not realistic.

17. How do other disciplines handle the integration of research into practice?

It varies with the setting. University-affiliated settings have more structured approaches—journal clubs, research committees, and other mechanisms. Often clinical research is an integral part of university-affiliated settings.

Many facilities that are not formally associated with universities provide clinical experience sites for students in medicine, pharmacy, nursing, and allied health professions and occupations. The faculty of these schools are an often untapped resource for research findings. If your facility has affiliations for student clinical experience, I encourage you to explore approaches to involve faculty in strengthening evidence-based practice.

Many facilities conduct grand rounds sessions that present research findings both in relation to a particular case and more generally in relation to particular conditions and treatments. Vendors of pharmaceuticals and medical products often sponsor speakers who address research findings related to, but not necessarily to endorse, the company's products.

Organizations' initiatives in organizational performance improvement, benchmarking, risk management, and quality improvement often incorporate relevant research findings in selecting new approaches to improving care.

There are many resources available to highlight relevant research. But in order for research findings to be consistently incorporated, someone or some group within the organization needs to make it happen:

- by formalizing and enforcing the requirement of including research findings where indicated, for example in inservice presentations and quality improvement recommendations
- by identifying and accessing appropriate potential resources for research findings

18. I always thought of research as looking up information about a particular topic in reference books, journals, and other sources (now including the Internet). Is that the type of evidence that is considered evidence-based practice?

Often the word "research" is used to describe the process of gathering information about a particular topic—anything from a personal purchase to very specific clinical issues. Strictly speaking, "conducting research" usually means planning and implementing controlled data collection, analyzing and interpreting the results, and drawing conclusions.

However, researching a topic, a medical product, or clinical approach can mean collecting information from various sources: publications, Internet sources, experts, vendors of products/pharmaceuticals, and perhaps others. This process is similar to the review of the literature in formal research. Having collected the information, you then critique the findings, synthesize, and apply what you have learned to the problem at hand.

Whether applying the information constitutes evidence-based practice really depends upon the credibility of your sources and how closely your practice situation parallels the settings and populations described in the information you collect.

19. Where do we look for research findings?

In this age of information, I hesitate to make specific suggestions because new resources become available almost daily. An important part of the evidence-based attitude is to continually search for new sources—via World Wide Web search engines, such as pubmed (**www.pubmedcentral.nih.gov**). Discovering new journals and other resources through sharing with staff is another possible source.

However, I can recommend a few credible sources:

- **www.ngc.gov**—evidence-based guidelines produced by the Agency for Healthcare Research and Quality (AHRQ), National Guideline Clearinghouse
- **www.cochrane.mcmaster.ca**—Cochrane Collaboration
- **www.acponline.org**—American College of Physicians Journal Club
- **www.cochrane.mcmaster.ca**—Best Evidence Data Base, McMaster University, Hamilton, Ontario
- *Evidence-Based Nursing*—a Canadian/United Kingdom publication begun in 1997
- *Critical Care Nurse*—has a feature, "Protocols for Practice"
- *Nursing Research*
- *Journal of Advanced Nursing*
- Web sites of specialty nursing professional organizations
- Web sites of schools of nursing that have ongoing research programs in particular specialty areas, such as the University of Iowa for gerontological nursing research

20. Are there applicable findings in research other than research related directly to clinical care?

Absolutely! Research that documents outcomes related to staffing is an example. The American Nurses Association (ANA) sponsors many such studies and makes findings available in written publications and at the Web site (**www.ana.org**). Recently reported studies (Aiken et al., 2001; Aiken et al., 2002; Needleman et al., 2002) link positive patient outcomes to RN staffing. Houser's (2000) research program focused on variables in staffing and their relationship to patient outcomes.

Similarly, the findings of studies in quality improvement, management, and other dimensions of healthcare form a relevant evidence-based foundation for creating an optimal environment for clinical care.

Resources

Aiken, L. H., Clarke, S. P., Sloane, D. M., Sochalski, J. A., Busse, R., Clarke, H., Giovannetti, P., Hunt, J., Rafferty, A. M., & Shamian, J. (2001). Nurses report on hospital care in five countries. *Health Affairs, 20*(3), 43–53.

Aiken, L. H., Clarke, S. P., Sloane, D. M., Sochalski, J. A., & Silber, J. H. (2002). Hospital staffing and patient mortality, nurse burnout and job dissatisfaction. *Journal of the American Medical Association, 288*(16), 1987–1993.

Alfaro-LeFevre, R. (2003). *Critical thinking in nursing: A practical approach* (3rd ed.). Philadelphia: Saunders.

Benner, P. (1989). *From novice to expert.* Menlo Park, CA: Addison-Wesley.

del Bueno, D. (1990). Evaluation: Myths, mysteries and obsessions. *Journal of Nursing Administration, 20*(11), 4–7.

Gennaro, S. (1994). Research utilization: An overview. *Journal of Obstetric, Gynecologic, and Neonatal Nursing, 23*, 313–319.

Hadwiger, S. (1999). Cultural competence case scenarios for critical care nursing education. *Nurse Educator, 24*(5), 47–51.

Houser, J. L. (2000). An evaluation of the relationship of the context of nursing care and patient outcomes. *Quest for Quality* sponsored by Mayo Continuing Nursing Education. November 4, 2001.

Hunt, J. (1981). Indicators for nursing practice: The use of research findings. *Journal of Advanced Nursing, 6*, 189–194.

Ingersoll, G. L. (2000). Evidence-based nursing: What it is and what it isn't. *Nursing Outlook, 48*, 151–152.

Kim, M. (2000). Connecting knowledge to practice: Evidence-based nursing. *Chart, 97*(9), 1, 4–6. (Journal of the Illinois Nurses Association)

Kim, M. (2000). Transferring knowledge to practice nursing. *Chart, 97*(9), 2. (Journal of the Illinois Nurses Association)

Kirkpatrick, D. L. (1971). *A practical guide for supervisory training and development.* Reading, MA: Addison-Wesley.

Needleman, J., Buerhaus, P., Mattke, S., Stewart, M., & Zelevinsky, K. (2002). Nurse staffing levels and the quality of care in hospitals. *New England Journal of Medicine, 346*, 1715–1722.

Perry, K. (2000). The evidence is in: Let's use it. *Chart, 97*(9), 5–6. (Journal of the Illinois Nurses Association)

Tanner, C. (1999). Evidence-based practice: Research and critical thinking. *Journal of Nursing Education, 38*(3), 99.

Ulsenheimer, J., Bailey, D. McCullough, E., Thornton, S., & Warden, E. (1997). Thinking about thinking. *The Journal of Continuing Education in Nursing, 28*(4), 150–156.

Wynd, C. (2002). Evidence-based education and the evaluation of a critical care course. *The Journal of Continuing Education in Nursing, 33*(3), 119–125.

Chapter 16: Research and the Role of Critical Thinking and Clinical Judgment

"Discovery consists of seeing what everybody has seen and thinking what nobody has thought."

—Albert Szent-Gyorgyi de Nagyraolt, 1893–1986, American biochemist, 1937 Nobel Prize, "consummate scientist"

1. Why is critical thinking so important to research?

In my experience critical thinking is integral to the research process through proactive planning, creativity, and flexibility in designing the study and discriminating and analyzing current literature. Flexibility and perseverance are part of the process as well when faced with challenges and logical reasoning and are fundamental to analyzing outcomes. I had the privilege of working as a student nurse research assistant with Donna Wong, Kristi Nix, and Lynn Clutter, on their work refining the descriptors for the *Wong-Baker FACES Scale* for pain. I observed critical thinking skills and behaviors among these professionals which included meticulous attention to detail, flexibility when faced with on-site testing challenges, and proactive planning of data analysis prior to collecting data.

Collaboration among team members was evident as they worked to overcome challenges faced at different testing sites. The team persevered to continue to improve the pain scale and carefully document their research process so the pain scale's use in practice would be continually improved with the hopes of transforming nursing and improving patient outcomes. Their commitment to the integrity of the process, and the need to clearly identify any weaknesses in the study were essential components of the success of their project.

The characteristics of critical thinking are consistent with my lived experience of working with proficient researchers. Expert researchers are successful, in my opinion, because they demonstrate consistency with the consensus statement on critical thinking in nursing (Scheffer & Rubenfeld, 2000). It is clear to me that in the systematic process of research, those "ten habits of the mind and seven skills," are the same ingredients in the research process itself (see Table 16.1). I could not imagine conducting research without any one of these components.

TABLE 16.1 Essentials of Critical Thinking

Habits of Mind	Critical Thinking Skills
contextual perspective	analyzing
confidence	applying standards
creativity	discriminating
flexibility	information seeking
inquisitiveness	logical reasoning
intellectual integrity	predicting knowledge
intuition	transforming knowledge
open-mindedness	
perseverance	
reflection	

2. Is critical thinking part of the research process, and if so, in what way?

Critical thinking is an integral part of the research process as the researcher plans, thinks proactively, and integrates past experience with scholarly knowledge and a scientific approach. The researcher must be creative if stumbling blocks appear or a rewrite of the research question is in order.

The blend of knowledge, experience, expertise, flexibility, insight, and reflection is integral for critical thinking in research. Critical thinking can be defined many ways, which led one researcher to investigate definitions of critical thinking. Gordon (2000) conducted a study entitled "Congruency in defining critical thinking by nurse educators and non-nurse scholars" and found researching to be included in the definition of critical thinking by nurse educators. In addition to researching, nurse educators listed other characteristics of critical thinking including problem solving, decision making, and planning as integral to the definition of critical thinking.

3. What exactly is the research process?

Nursing research is as traditional as Florence Nightingale who collected data in a systematic way and implemented changes in practice based on the trends she observed in the data (a real critical thinker!). The nursing research process itself actually took off in the 1950s (Doordan, 1998). Doordan explained the research process as being:

- Systematic
- Purposeful

- An approach to gather information
- Used to describe information
- Evaluated for importance
- Carefully planned—including planning how to analyze data prior to beginning to collect the data

The process involves these steps:

1. Begin with an idea or a question to validate
2. Explore through a literature review
3. Summarize literature review
4. Define variables
5. Decide on method for study/qualitative/quantitative, mixed methodology
6. Collect data carefully
7. Review data critically
8. Analyze and summarize data
9. Disseminate information for use in practice/education/further research

You will note that many of these points are similar to Table 16.1 describing critical thinking skills and habits of mind, making the two processes an obvious connection. In short, it all begins with an idea, followed by data, and ends with what you do with that data to make "sense" out of it.

4. So, where do I begin the research process?

Begin with the concept or topic you are passionate about. Conduct a thorough literature review of research studies related to your area of interest and see whose names reappear on the searches. A researcher may have conducted multiple studies looking at various aspects of the concept. So, read a variety of studies and prepare to analyze them.

Use your critical thinking skills to evaluate the concepts and see if the definitions are clear and thoroughly defined. Read the purpose of the study, and if it is a quantitative study, make sure the variables are measurable, and the sample size is large enough to measure the targeted population. If it is a qualitative study, evaluate if the process was logical and if conclusions were consistent with the information collected.

Be sure to read the outcomes to see if they relate to the purpose. It is amazing to read published studies and find the outcomes and conclusions have no relation to what was described in the purpose. Keep your eyes open for clarity, precision, and accuracy. The literature review and critical evaluation of published research in your area of interest can be the springboard to narrowing the concept in preparation for beginning the research process. If you are an undergraduate or graduate student, be sure to follow the guidelines given to you by your professor. I know it sounds obvious, but this tidbit can be a lifesaver.

5. What do I do if I need advice on how to proceed with the research process?

If you know a professor who has experience with research, go and seek advice. If you are unsure who could provide guidance and perhaps even mentorship, start by talking to the dean of the local school of nursing or health sciences, a clinical nurse specialist, or the staff educator. If you are a student, go to a professor during office hours or make an appointment to discuss the research proposal. Many mentor/mentee relationships start as teacher/student relationships and can be mutually beneficial.

As an adjunct professor myself, I am amazed at how few students come in during the professor's office hours for guidance on their research or research proposal. Most professors are willing to talk through difficulties and provide reassurance or guidance. Sometimes the proposal needs clarity, or the student has set up the methodology and tools in a way that the data obtained will be meaningless. Be willing to talk to a statistics expert if necessary. Most undergraduate and graduate programs offer referrals (usually free) to a statistics expert located in the institution. Statistics experts may not know the topic, but they help you design a way to measure your ideas. Early guidance from your professor or a mentor, following written guidelines, and a statistics consult can help make the research proposal and subsequent research more meaningful. For qualitative research, pairing with an experienced qualitative researcher has proved invaluable for many novice researchers. Again, a dean or faculty member at a local school of nursing should be able to provide assistance.

6. How can I get some ideas about research topics?

A good place to spend some time is the Web site at the National Institutes of Health (NIH); read about current nursing research, who the researchers are, what are they studying, and what areas of research they are interested in pursuing in the future. The NIH Web site is located at **http://www.nih.gov**; you can search for topics and principle researchers on the link CRISP. The research link that is discipline specific for the National Institute for Nursing Research (NINR) is associated with the NIH and located at **http://www. nih.gov/ninr/**.

The NINR has a link on its Web site entitled "call for papers," which is an excellent way to narrow your topic and look for areas needing further investigation.

7. How can I gain experience in research?

Ask the dean of the local school of nursing for information on current nursing research being conducted in the area. Frequently, as in my case, an experienced researcher will allow students interested in pursuing research to assist with the research process, collecting data, or other tasks. It is invaluable experience to work with a nurse researcher actively involved in a research project. Another way is to apply for the American Association of Critical Care Nurses (AACN) mentorship grant, which will not only provide funding but support for a novice researcher by being paired with an experienced researcher in the novice's area of interest. You can find out more at the Web site **www.aacn.org**; click on "clinical practice" and then on "research."

8. Are there any good written resources for research?

Here are three of the best books, which I highly recommend. If you need guidance in understanding critical thinking and how to apply critical thinking concepts, I recommend *Clinical Reasoning: The Art and Science of Critical and Creative Thinking* by Daniel J. Pesut and JoAnne Herman (1999), published by Delmar. For practical tips I recommend *Research Survival Guide* by Ann Marttinen Doordan (1998), published by Lippincott. Another excellent book is *Research Strategies for Clinicians* by Bradi B. Granger and Marianne Chulay (1999), published by Appleton and Lange.

On the Internet, you will find a wealth of information on the Web site for Sigma Theta Tau, the International Nursing Honor Society, and you do not have to be a member to enjoy some of the many benefits. The home-page is at **www. nursingsociety.org**; click on research for several helpful tools and articles. The newer Web site (**www.nursinglibrary.org**) is the *Online Journal of Knowledge Synthesis for Nursing* which has free educational articles as well as the opportunity to subscribe to the journal.

9. How do I find funding for my research?

Good question. Grants and funding are available, and most schools of nursing can provide written literature on available funding, so ask. Another good source of available grant information is the American Association of Critical Care

Nurses. You can log on to the Web site at **http://www.aacn.org** or call the AACN 1-800-394-5995, ext. 377, or you may send an e-mail to AACN for more information (e-mail **research@aacn.org**). Also, the **http://www.nih.gov** Web site of the NIH contains helpful links for finding grants and funding for research.

10. I've completed my research; how do I get published?

Terrific question! It is always exciting to have your hard work recognized and published. The AACN provides a program called the AACN Wyeth-Ayerst Fellows Program designed to pair an experienced mentor with the novice for the purpose of developing written work for publication in a professional journal. Call the AACN number listed above for more information on the Fellows program.

Another possibility is to obtain publication guidelines from journals known to publish research such as *Nursing Research* or *The Journal of Nursing Scholarship*, the journal of the nursing honor society Sigma Theta Tau International, and submit your manuscript for review.

11. Are there any current studies that I could use to relate the effectiveness of critical thinking to clinical practice?

DiVito Thomas (2000) recently completed her dissertation, a mixed methodology research study investigating critical thinking and clinical nursing judgment. Her results were statistically significant. You may contact her for more information regarding her critical thinking research at **pdvthomas@oru.edu**.

Also, Robert Bienkowski has an interesting proposal you can read on the Web site for the National Institute of Nursing Research at **http://www.nih.gov/ninr/**. Search the CRISP section for grant number 1R13HS01958 and principle investigator Robert Bienkowski for his proposed research conference "Utilizing research to enhance clinical practice." The goal of the conference is aimed at influencing patient care by increasing evidence-based practice.

12. How would I get started if I wanted to conduct such a study?

Begin by listing your areas of interest and what you could investigate to enhance your clinical practice. For example, Ptlene Minick researched an area of crucial importance to critical care nurses, advanced cardiac life support (ACLS) knowledge. Her study was published in the March/April 1996 issue of *Journal of Nursing Staff Development*. In it, she recommended mock codes as often as every six months for nurses to retain the crucial ACLS information.

Find a topic that interests you and plan a project to answer the question of how it relates to clinical practice and enhances critical thinking by nurses. Again, check the Web site for the National Institute of Nursing Research at **http://www.nih.gov/ninr/** to review the current topics listed under investigation for ideas.

13. If I were to support staff in a research project in a department, or on a unit, what are some pointers for getting started?

Always capitalize on the staff expertise available in the unit; recognize their clinical knowledge; recruit their assistance; and reward and recognize their participation and input. Once you have lined out the topic, question, methodology, instruments, and methods of statistical analysis, use staff for data collection.

Be sure to obtain approval in writing. Decide if you will need to create a patient consent form and if so, you will need approval from the institutional review board to ensure patient confidentiality and safety. If in doubt how to start, contact a local school of nursing and inquire as to the possibility of a nursing faculty acting as a sponsor/mentor for the project.

If you are having difficulty obtaining approval from nursing leadership or the institutional review board, recruit key nurses to assist you in revising the proposal and/or in helping you get a meeting with the appropriate research approval committees. Make sure all responsibilities are clearly defined, costs estimated, and deadlines for data collection settled upon.

14. How can I show support of the development of critical thinking in terms of research?

Conduct a search of current literature on CINAHL, the Cumulative Index to Nursing and Allied Health Literature at **www.cinahl.com**, or the National Institute of Nursing Research Web site and read the current studies published by nurse researchers on the topic of critical thinking.

15. Are there any creative ideas for connecting the development of critical thinking with a research project?

Yes! A group of researchers (Parker & Minick, 1999) decided to look at the clinical decision making by a group of expert perioperative nurses. They found intricate patterns of concern, assessment, and caring. This was a very creative way to study the impact RNs make on clinical practice.

16. I would love to have the staff more involved in researching nursing practice, and I think the link between the two could be motivating. What do you think?

Excellent idea! At the next staff meeting have nurses brainstorm on areas of practice in the unit that you would like to affect. Develop priorities and tackle them one at a time. See if you can develop a nursing research committee and conduct the research under the guidance of a master's prepared (or higher, if available) nurse educator or Clinical Nurse Specialist and channel that enthusiasm into an insightful, meaningful, nursing research project that becomes part of your identity as a unit—the unit that integrates research and practice! Again, if you need guidance, check the AACN Web site for ideas and read a good book like *Research Strategies for Clinicians* by Bradi B. Granger and Marianne Chulay, Appleton & Lange, 1999.

This book has step-by-step instructions for beginning a research project and is written in user-friendly terms. For example:

- Beginning the journey: improving patient outcomes using research
- Tools to measure outcomes
- Brainstorming high-volume patient care issues
- Identification of potential research topics or questions
- Examining clinical pathways for variances or complications
- Using national and regional benchmark data
- Using research priorities identified by professional associations
- Prioritizing clinical questions
- Institutional priorities
- Cost issues
- Cost evaluation worksheet
- Research teams: getting started, keeping momentum
- Team roles and responsibilities
- Dealing with conflict and communicating within and beyond the team
- Pragmatic approaches to literature reviews, first, second, and third rounds
- Protocol development: keep-it-simple strategies for the novice and the expert
- Draft mode
- Linking data collection to data form and databases
- Getting through the approval process

- Contracts and agreements
- Data analysis
- Sharing your findings
- Finding resources to support research
- Examples of Institutional Review Board (IRB) forms

17. What examples of possible research outcomes would help me put together a project with advanced practice nurses who want to demonstrate autonomy in decision making?

Excellent question. If they are really serious, there is a Web site at the National Institute of Nursing Research on becoming a nursing research scientist (**http://ninr.cm.net/**). Several studies investigating advanced practice nurse autonomy are listed such as "Diffusion and Sustainability of Nurse-Managed Practices" by Linda Campbell. You might also want to check out another study listed on the National Institute for Nursing Research Web site conducted by Marie Cowan entitled "Care Management by Nurse Practitioner/Hospitalist Team." By investigating current studies, the advanced practice nurses may find inspiration for launching their own study on autonomy. For example, Karen Kelly Schutzenhofer and Donna Bridgman Musser (1994) conducted the nurse autonomy study. The descriptive study discovered significant relationships between autonomy and five characteristics such as age, work experience, education, organizational membership, gender-stereotyped personality traits and professional nursing autonomy. The researchers used valid and reliable tools and found that nurses with their position or title as a CNS (clinical nurse specialist) or NP (nurse practitioner) had significantly higher nursing activity traits than either managers or staff nurses. You may read more about this study at the Sigma Theta Tau International Web site (**www.nursinglibrary.org**).

18. Any last advice?

Keep your focus, accept peer and expert review of your work, seek excellence, accept constructive criticism, and use your research to enhance nursing practice. Remember, the research process is akin to embarking on a journey. Some stages in the research process are predictable and planned, such as obtaining approval, or undergoing institutional review, or evaluating outcomes. However, you may have surprises along the way and have to adjust your itinerary, shift your priorities, or choose a slightly different path. Most undergraduate programs and master's level programs require a research class or two and either completion of a research proposal or a research project. Keep your passion, your vision, and enthusiasm. Seek encouragement and support from peers and experienced researchers. The journey alone is worth your efforts, and just think, your research could influence future nursing practices.

RESOURCES

Beecroft, P., & Lindquist, R. (Eds.). (1995). *Writing a successful research grant proposal: A beginner's guide.*

Alisa Viejo, CA: American Association of Critical-Care Nurses.

DiVito Thomas, P. (2000). Identifying critical thinking behaviors in clinical judgments. *Journal for Nurses in Staff Development, 16*(4), 174–180.

Doordan, A. M. (1998). *Lippincott's need-to-know: Research survival guide*. Philadelphia: Lippincott.

Gordon, J. M. (2000). Congruency in defining critical thinking by nurse educators and non-nurse scholars. *Journal of Nursing Education, 39*(8), 338–339.

Granger, B., & Chulay, M. (1999). *Research strategies for clinicians*. Stamford, CT: Appleton & Lange.

Nix, K., Clutter, L., & Wong, D. (1993). *The influence of type of instructions in measuring pain in young children using the FACES Pain rating scale*. Unpublished research study. Information available online (**http://www.us.elsevierhealth.com/WOW/facesResearch.html**).

O'Steen, D. S., Kee, C. C., & Minick, P. (1996). The retention of advanced cardiac life support knowledge among registered nurses. *Journal of Nursing Staff Development, 12*(2), 66–72.

Parker, C., & Minick, P. (1999). Clinical decision-making processes in perioperative nursing. *Journal of the Association of Operating Room Nurses, 70*(1), 45–48.

Scheffer, B. K., & Rubenfeld, M. G. (2000). A consensus statement on critical thinking in nursing. *Journal of Nursing Education, 39*(8), 352–359.

Schutzenhofer, K. K., & Musser, D. (1994). Nurse characteristics and professional autonomy. *Image: Journal of Nursing Scholarship, 26*(3), 201–205.

Section 4:

Appreciating the Benefits of the Elephant's Work: Attracting, Developing, and Maintaining the Best Critical Thinkers on the Clinical Team

The previous sections have focused on developing critical thinking students and staff. This section looks at how we can retain our best staff thinkers so they can help lead the clinical team. Managers, educators, and coworkers share in the responsibility of team development.

17. Staff Satisfaction and Critical Thinking

Donna Ignatavicius, MS, RN

18. Recruitment and Retention

Donna Ignatavicius, MS, RN
Bette Case, PhD, RN, BC
Marilynn Jackson, PhD, MA, RN

Chapter 17: Staff Satisfaction and Critical Thinking

"Pleasure in the job puts perfection in the work."

—Aristotle, 384–322 BC

1. What are the main reasons why nursing retention is so poor around the country?

Several issues may give us some insight into why retention in many healthcare settings is low. I should mention to you, though, that some places aren't really having a problem with nurse retention. So, what we need to do is see what they're doing right, and how it may be different from what your agency is doing. I can always tell when I go into a hospital whether there's a high or low retention rate. It's often related to the organizational culture and morale. If nurses feel valued, they'll stay; if they don't, they're going to leave.

If you recall, in a previous chapter (Chapter 9, Question 18), I discussed the success of "magnet" hospitals in recruiting and retaining nurses. And the good news is that the number of magnet hospitals in which nurses are empowered to be a vital part of the organization decision-making process is continuing to grow (Gasda, 2002). For an updated list of those hospitals, see **www.nursingworld.org/ancc/magnet**.

We know that nurses want to give the best possible care that they can. When nurses perceive barriers that prevent them from giving that level of care, they become very frustrated. Some of the barriers that I have heard nurses talk about and are validated in the literature are listed in Table 17.1.

The best approach is to assess which barriers you might have in your organization, and try to find ways to overcome them. For instance, if nurses are hesitant or unsure about how to delegate and supervise, they need to be taught and then have an opportunity to practice this process with a mentor.

2. Then, do you have any suggestions about how to keep nurses on medical-surgical units?

I think the most important approach is to determine what medical-surgical nurses want. In other words, what keeps them satisfied, and what are the dissatisfiers. What about patient load? Do they have ample time to provide quality care? What barriers in Table 17.1 are they dealing with? Are there ways to overcome them?

TABLE 17.1 Perceived Barriers to Providing Quality Patient Care

- Shortage of professional nurses
- Too much time spent on non-nursing tasks, such as transporting patients and delivering meal trays
- Increase in unlicensed assistive personnel (UAP)
- Lack of knowledge about how to delegate and supervise UAP
- Lack of adequate training for UAP
- Inadequate preparation for professional practice
- Lack of mentors or role models
- Lack of empowerment to make decisions that affect the organization
- Lack of empowerment to make decisions regarding patient care
- Conflicts with physicians regarding the most appropriate patient care
- Focus of the organization on costs and the "bottom line"

3. We've had a hard time recruiting staff because we compete with several other agencies. Recruitment bonuses just don't seem to be that helpful. Any ideas?

Recruitment bonuses are only a short-term fix. Sure, it's fairly easy to attract nurses for money, but will they stay? I think we should be focusing more attention on retention efforts—perhaps even retention bonuses. Several hospitals do give additional monies to nurses who stay a certain length of time, and continue to reward them in this way.

The key to retention, of course, is to find out what nurses want—what are the satisfiers for them, what keeps them with the organization. And, conversely, what are the dissatisfiers? If they outweigh what the nurses want, then they'll leave. Most nurses realize that you can't please everyone and all of their dissatisfiers may not go away. But, listening to their concerns and giving them feedback makes nurses feel that someone is listening.

4. Frequently, clinical unit educators and clinical specialists have to pitch in to help with staffing. But then, they don't get a chance to do their jobs adequately. How can we prevent this problem?

This may not be a problem, but an opportunity. While it may seem that educators and CNSs aren't getting "their" jobs done, in fact, they are validating their functions. By working with the staff, more cooperative relationships can be established, needs assessments can be validated, and just-in-time training can be provided. A periodic check to see how often this occurs may help to maintain roles.

5. Doesn't critical thinking relate to staff satisfaction and retention?

In my opinion, yes. We know that if nurses have a say in how staffing problems will be resolved and how nursing care will be delivered, they'll be happier. Overall, nurses have good critical thinking skills and they can come up with possible solutions for staffing crises and other problems within the nursing department.

6. Some nurses tell me that they want to have a say in the decisions here. But when they have an idea and use their critical thinking skills, they are sometimes discouraged by their peers, and sometimes even the physicians. How do I deal with that?

I think that in some places, critical thinking is risk-taking. Yet, how will things get changed if someone is not willing to take a risk? I believe that most nurses will stand up for what they believe in. And, what they believe in is quality patient care. We are advocates for patients, and we know that inadequate staffing leads to errors and poor patient outcomes, including increased deaths.

Fortunately, most physicians view us as valuable, professional colleagues. We have to stay knowledgeable, though, and behave professionally when we approach them.

7. Some nurses don't seem to want to contribute to new ideas. How do we motivate them?

How do we motivate people to do anything? How do we convince people to stop smoking or drinking? If they don't value *not* smoking or drinking as much as they do enjoying these habits, then they won't stop. Valuing a behavior is the key to motivation.

I think this analogy tells us that nurses have to value the experience of coming up with new ideas and critically thinking. It does take energy to think. I often hear nurses say that they've contributed ideas, but they were "put down" or they were never told why the idea wasn't accepted. After a while, they simply give up because they think that "nothing's going to change anyway. So, why bother?"

The message, then, is that nurses have to have an outlet where they can contribute ideas to the decision making of the organization, and then receive timely feedback about where those ideas are. I'm not sure if managers and other nursing leaders are as diligent as they should be when it comes to providing timely feedback. But, they need to be!

8. The case managers are complaining that nurses don't focus on patient outcomes for discharge. They just seem to be more concerned about getting through their day. Is that a common problem?

Case management is often viewed by bedside nursing staff as a process in which case managers spend a lot of time on the phone with third party payers, and the rest of their time doing discharge planning. And, that's because the case management model used in many places is just that—utilization management and discharge planning. If case managers were really looking at the continuum of care on a daily basis and working more closely with the staff, nurses would have a better understanding and appreciation for their role.

All members of the healthcare team, including the case manager, are supposed to be focused on the same outcomes for patients and residents. So, everyone needs to be "walking the talk." I'd like to see more dialogue between nursing and case management, and a better explanation to nurses how they can help patients achieve positive outcomes. Sometimes figuring out how to achieve those outcomes takes a collaborative critical thinking approach.

9. Why aren't nurses more interdisciplinary care focused?

We've been taught for many years that we are in a unique profession. And to some extent, I think that's true. However, we still must learn how to work within the healthcare system framework and how to collaborate more effectively. In most nursing programs, there's very little or no opportunity to do that. I believe that needs to change. As part of their clinical time, students need an opportunity to work with other disciplines on a more personal level.

10. How can we get nurses and other healthcare professionals to focus more on expected outcomes and collaborate with other healthcare team members?

This requires knowledge of outcomes and the contributions of the healthcare team members. Facilitating a conversation with the pharmacist, role modeling addressing the social worker, and rehearsing a challenge with a physician can be helpful strategies.

Using standardized nursing language, such as Nursing Outcomes Classification (2000) can help teach staff how to focus on outcomes. Care maps and critical pathways had the right idea but require our expertise to make them realistic and manageable. It takes a constant focus on outcomes with frequent facilitation to achieve success.

11. Some nurses don't attend continuing education opportunities, go back for degrees, or read any journal articles. Isn't there a relationship between knowledge and critical thinking?

One of the characteristics of a critical thinker is that the individual must be knowledgeable. And, healthcare knowledge is changing all the time. If we don't have knowledgeable nurses, they can't possibly use critical thinking to its fullest extent. It's hard to think about what you don't know!

12. But, some nurses complain that they don't have time to read journals. Things are changing so rapidly, and I know everyone needs to keep up. So, how can I help them to continue their learning?

One way to keep up with journals is to establish an online journal club. Ask several nurses on a unit or department to volunteer to read at least one article out of the current month's journals. Then, each volunteer summarizes the article in several sentences and puts the synopsis on e-mail for all staff. I also prefer if the volunteers add a sentence about how they think the staff can incorporate the information into daily practice. In some cases, there's a need to change nursing policies and procedures based on new evidence-based information. These articles and their implications can be discussed in staff meetings.

An example of what a nurse might write about an article follows in Table 17.2.

TABLE 17.2   Example of Article Summary and Implications for Nursing Practice

D'Arcy, Y. (2002). How to treat arthritis pain. *Nursing, 32*(7), 30–31.
The American Pain Society (APA) recently published new guidelines for managing pain in patients with osteoarthritis (OA) and rheumatoid arthritis (RA). For mild OA, use acetaminophen (Tylenol); for more severe OA pain, give a COX–2 NSAID, such as rofecoxib (Vioxx).
For patients with RA, treat with disease-modifying drugs, such as methotrexate (Trexall) or leflunomide (Arava). For pain, use COX–2 NSAIDs. Opioids may be used only for patients who do not respond to these drugs.
Implications for nursing practice. We need to be aware of these evidence-based guidelines and question physicians who do not appropriately prescribe according to these guidelines. Also, the Pain Management Committee needs to educate physicians and other prescribers about arthritis pain management to standardize and assure best practices.

Another method for ongoing education is weekly clinical teaching rounds. Clinical rounds provide onsite continuous learning and professional growth, while taking little time to implement (Guin, Connelly, & Briggs, 2002). These learning experiences help develop critical thinking skills if the rounds leader poses questions that help nurses see a holistic approach to patient care.

13. I've been hearing a lot about those terms—"best practices" and "evidence-based practice." What exactly do these terms mean?

Best practices are the best possible care that can be given to a patient. How do we know if we're providing the best possible care? Because we keep up with the latest research, guidelines (like the pain guidelines in Table 17.2), and standards of care that have been established by authoritative and professional healthcare groups. These sources of information are called the "evidence;" thus, the term evidence-based practice (Hamer & Collinson, 1999). Chapter 15 discusses these concepts in detail.

14. How do I implement evidence-based nursing practice in an agency?

It's difficult if nurses aren't interested in learning and examining their practice to ensure that they are incorporating current knowledge. They have to be motivated and guided in this process. What will they get out of it? What will patients get out of it? As I said earlier, they have to value evidence-based practice (EBP) before they will make an attempt to examine their practices.

15. What barriers should we expect as we attempt to implement evidence-based practice?

A few common barriers are listed in Table 17.3 below.

Remember that you shouldn't wait until everyone is ready. The rule of thumb is that if a third or more of the nurses are behind a potential change or process, proceed. Many others will join later, and a few will be outliers and either try to

TABLE 17.3 Barriers to Implementing Evidence-Based Practice in Nursing

• Don't like or understand research	• Apathetic; lack energy
• Satisfied with the status quo	• Patients are satisfied now, so why change anything?
• Fear of the unknown	• Possibly more work
• Need for further education	• Lack of readily available resources

sabotage the plan or not participate. It's up to leadership to hold these nurses accountable for best practices. If they're not performing at the desired level, they may need disciplinary action, which could include negative consequences.

16. How do we deal with those few physicians who continue to practice the same way for years, and refuse to change?

Schools of medicine are changing their approach to teaching and learning, making this problem disappear eventually. In the meantime, using a consistent and respectful approach can be most helpful.

Introducing new ideas can be difficult and may require repetition. For example, if the physician continues to order only a PT for Coumadin management rather than the INR, and this is a problem, then perhaps the laboratory and the pharmacy can offer educational sessions on these topics to the nurses. The fliers can be helpful if placed in the physicians' work area or sent to the specific physician. The department chair or performance improvement department may support a change in practice by directly speaking to the physician.

Carefully weighing what has to be changed because it is a significant improvement with what's not can be tough. Look at all we've learned about cholesterol through the years. However, solid information with sound reasoning that helps patients is hard to argue with. Find an ally and together deliver the information and give enough time for the physician to change his/her practice in his/her own terms.

17. What resources will we need to implement evidence-based practice?

The resources that are needed appear in Table 17.4 below.

It's especially important that all of these resources be readily available to staff at all levels. In some facilities, only the managers and educators have Internet

TABLE 17.4   Resources Needed to Implement Evidence-Based Practice (EBP) in Nursing

• Internet access	• Current printed references, including textbooks
• Current journals	
• Adequate staff to implement EBP	• Time to plan and implement changes
• Open communication	• Strong quality improvement program
• Advanced practice nurses who can interpret research findings	• Teamwork and collaboration

and journal access. A central library is often not staffed, and if it is, the hours it is open may not coincide with the nurses' hours of work.

18. How do we mesh evidence-based practice with the current orientation program?

It really doesn't take more time to incorporate information about EBP into orientation. Simply ensure that you are giving new (and experienced) nurses the most current information available, and that policies and procedures reflect the most current research. Another tip is that I think we sometimes present information and add that it is a Joint Commission on Accreditation of Healthcare Organizations (JCAHO) requirement, as if that's the only reason to provide good care. Instead, stress the need to do "X" is because it's the right thing to do—it's based on current evidence!

19. How do I convince administration that we need to refocus on professional practice and increase learning opportunities for nurses? Education costs money!

Data speak volumes. Find a small success where a simple intervention reduced length of stay, cost, or mortality, or suggest the use of an evidence-based practice guideline and share the positive results experienced by other facilities. If the focus was cost, inquire about what changes contributed to the decreased learning opportunities. Was your predecessor ineffective? Was the previous administrator a lawyer rather than a clinician? Is there a corporate superstructure? Did staff abuse their educational leave time? The solution may be unrelated to the apparent dissatisfying problem. Partner with administration. Seek clarification on the vision and goals and demonstrate how education can save money.

RESOURCES

Gasda, K. A. (2002). The magnetic pull. *Nursing Management, 33*(4), 45–46.

Guin, P., Counsell, C. M., & Briggs, S. (2002). Round out your department. *Nursing Management, 33*(5), 24.

Hamer, S., & Collinson, G. (1999). *Achieving evidence-based practice.* Edinburgh, UK: Bailliere-Tindall.

Johnson, M., Maas, M., & Moorhead, S. (2000). *Nursing Outcomes Classification.* St. Louis: Mosby.

Sedlak, C., & Doheny, M. (1998). Peer review through clinical rounds: A collaborative critical thinking strategy. *Nurse Educator, 23*(5), 42–45.

Chapter 18: Recruitment and Retention

> *"If you want to build a ship, don't drum up people together to collect wood and don't assign them tasks and work, but rather teach them to long for the endless immensity of the sea."*
>
> —Antoine de Saint-Exupery

1. I've heard that there's a relationship between critical thinking and staff recruitment/retention. I agree, but I'm curious what your perceptions are.

Most nurses value autonomy in their practice. Being autonomous entails the ability to make decisions that influence the direction of the organization/unit, as well as those that affect patient care. I've observed that organizations that foster and reward critical thinking attract the most qualified and dedicated nurses.

2. We talk a lot about wanting nurses to think critically, but it's not emphasized enough in what we do here. Any suggestions as to how to get started?

Critical thinking has to be formally recognized as a core value of the healthcare organization. The leadership then empowers nurses and other employees to critically think. Without administrative support, any other suggestions probably won't work. So, the first step is to get administrative buy in!

3. Shouldn't critical thinking be an expectation in job descriptions?

Of course, it should be. Some think that critical thinking is implied in their job descriptions and performance appraisals because they use the term nursing process. But, as you've read in Section 1 of this book, critical thinking is not the same as the nursing process—it is at a higher level of thinking, not linear steps of the problem-solving process.

The indicators and cognitive processes that were described in Section 1 and then referred to throughout this book provide lots of ideas about what should be in a job description to emphasize critical thinking. In Chapter 5, I also talked about emotional IQ skills that go hand-in-hand with critical thinking. For example, the professional nurse should be able to accurately and completely interpret assessment data. That is a higher level of cognition than just collecting pertinent patient data.

4. What is the difference between a job description and a role description?

According to the latest human resources literature, a job description focuses more on tasks, whereas a role description focuses more on outcomes. Job descriptions tend to be a laundry list of tasks and functions that are unrelated to the desired results or outcomes of the work. Role descriptions, on the other hand, focus on what outcomes the employee is expected to achieve, and hold the employee accountable for meeting them (Porter-O'Grady & Wilson, 1995). Table 18.1 further differentiates job and role descriptions.

5. I believe that preceptors need more training in how to develop critical thinking in orientees. How should we tackle this?

The two most important precepting strategies for teaching critical thinking are role modeling (accompanied by thinking-out-loud) and questioning. The preceptor as role model makes his/her thought process "visible" by pointing out to the orientee:

- What the preceptor observed that triggered the critical thinking process
- What additional information the preceptor needed to act
- How the preceptor interpreted the information
- How the preceptor chose the particular action

TABLE 18.1   Differentiating Between Jobs and Roles

Jobs	Roles
Specific, defined tasks and functions	Fluid and flexible guidelines
Task- and process-driven	Outcomes-driven
Based on specific criteria/events	Based on continuum of growth
Delegated functions	Inherent in role
Responsibilities outlined	Accountability emphasized

Note: From *The leadership revolution in health care: Altering systems, changing behaviors* (p. 209), by T. Porter-O'Grady and C. K. Wilson, 1995, Gaithersburg, MD: Aspen. Copyright 1995 by Aspen. Adapted with permission.

- How the preceptor evaluated and will continue to evaluate and monitor the efficacy of the chosen action
- Other critical thinking behaviors that the preceptor employs in particular situations

The point is that usually only the *results* of critical thinking are observable so the preceptor must make explicit the use of critical thinking behaviors.

The preceptor might also *ask* the orientee rather than tell the orientee—for example, "What additional information did I need before I could proceed?"

The preceptor's full range of questions includes those designed to evoke the critical thinking behaviors described elsewhere in this book. For example:

- What is the difference between the way Mr. Jones is responding to this drug and the way Mrs. Harris is responding? What is causing this difference?
- Who else do we need to get involved in making this decision?
- What's wrong with this picture?
- How is this procedure different from the way you did it at your previous job (or, for the new graduate, in school)?

These are only a few sample questions; the preceptor's goal is to ask questions that require the orientee to practice critical thinking. The questions which best evoke critical thinking require more than a "yes" or "no" answer and ask the orientee to describe his/her thinking.

6. We tell staff not to be task-oriented, but the competencies that we assess are mostly psychomotor skills. How do we decide what other skills to assess?

In each clinical unit, identify the nursing activities that meet these familiar Joint Commission on Accreditation of Healthcare Organizations (JCAHO)-mandated criteria:

- High frequency—that is, skills and judgments that come up very frequently
- High risk—skills and judgments that create safety risks for patients and/or others
- Problem-prone—skills and judgments that cause problems for nurses, patients, or others
- High risk, low volume—skills and judgments that are high risk and do not occur frequently enough for the nurse to practice regularly

7. Competent workers are the ones that we want to attract and to keep. What's the best method for assessing competencies?

The best method, and the method which JCAHO requires, is to document competency in the performance appraisal. Therefore, the assessment process should relate directly to performance appraisal criteria. In most organizations, this takes some fine tuning. Bear in mind the distinction between competence and competency. Competence refers to the knowledge base one needs for safe, legal, effective practice. Competence, therefore, might be tested on a written test. Competency refers to actual practice, drawing upon and using the knowledge base. Competencies are specific, discrete behavioral descriptions that sum to overall competency. It is essential that methods used to assess competence and competency replicate actual practice situations as closely as possible. This implies the use of simulations and perhaps audiotaped interactions, videotaped vignettes, computer-based situations or case studies, equipment displays to troubleshoot, and other relevant techniques that replicate practice.

You might present a series of situations that are described very briefly, perhaps in one or two sentences and ask the nurse a single question about all of the situations. That question might be "Is this safe or unsafe practice?" or "Is this documentation complete or incomplete?" or "Does that practice create a legal risk?" This method allows you to ask many questions that require the nurse to make judgments using a defined set of criteria (e.g., universal precautions, ethical standards). What makes this true-false style of questioning a critical thinking technique is that you are asking the nurse to make a judgment in a situation. Simply asking yes or no questions about what is or is not a part of a policy or procedure does not require judgment.

8. The educators and managers are part of the Nursing Standards Committee here. Sometimes I think that all of these policies and procedures limit critical thinking in staff. How can we address this issue?

The first question to be asked about making or revising any policy and procedure is "Do we need a policy for this?" The answer may be "yes" to protect patient safety, to improve efficiency, to ensure consistent high quality care, to prevent legal exposure, to satisfy accreditation requirements or perhaps for other reasons. There is no question that standardizing practice reduces risk of error. However, voluminous, complex policies and procedures create a risk of another kind—the risk of noncompliance. Policies and procedures provide legal and accreditation protection only when you can document that the policy and procedure have been followed. When policies and procedures become highly detailed they are likely to become obsolete more quickly. Nurses may even ignore complex policies and procedures and just "wing it."

Seek the counsel of the legal, quality, and risk management departments in the organization. Standards of practice of professional nursing organizations are also a useful resource. Policies and procedures should provide guidelines and criteria for safe, effective practice.

9. What is the liability if we make the policies with broader guidelines?

As mentioned previously, seek the counsel of the legal, quality, and risk management departments in the organization. Assure that you are protecting patient safety and that you are providing sufficient guidelines so that nurses are not wasting time figuring out how to do something when a simple guideline could improve safety, efficiency, and satisfaction. Preserve nurses' critical thinking energies for important clinical decisions by providing guidelines and resources.

10. Documentation takes up so much time, and reflects so little of what the nurses really do. How can an emphasis on critical thinking help?

The statistics regarding the hours of paperwork that are spent compared to the time spent in providing actual care support the nurses' views that charting is a time consuming and often thankless task. An article titled "Charting Critical Thinking" by Susan K. Chase, *Dimensions of Critical Care Nursing*, 1997, includes several examples of passive and active voice charting, recommending that we all consider including judgments about the data we are recording, as well as predictive and creative thoughts.

Consider the following example:

"Patient endoscoped in the unit in the AM and visited by sister from out of state during the PM. Tolerated weaning trial with no adverse effects, but appears less able to focus beyond himself this afternoon. Suggest shorter weaning period with longer rest on evenings. Observe closely tomorrow" (p. 105).

This brief progress note includes data, judgment, and plans for the future—a true representation of critical thinking, and it does not take an entire page!

11. Rehabilitation therapists consistently document patient progress toward expected outcomes on the medical record, but nurses document the things that we do. How do we get nurses to document progress toward outcomes?

As in discharge planning, the outcomes focus begins early in the relationship, and should start with some specific interview questions that ask the patient and/or family to identify the goals that they are working toward, either during the acute hospitalization, or for a longer term in a clinic setting, or a rehab area. Public and home health nurses take the lead here, having long ago determined that the results the patient and family hope to achieve are what drive the plan of care. Likewise, rehab nurses have adopted that approach, and it is second nature to look at both short and long term goals with the patient, and to document according to those. An interview/admission document that includes specific questions such as "What are your goals during this hospitalization?" or "What results can the healthcare team help you to achieve?" reinforces the emphasis on goals, and provides an opportunity for the discussion and the documentation of planned outcomes.

12. Is there a documentation system that would help nurses focus more on outcomes?

An Interdisciplinary Plan of Care (Figure 18-1) that begins with a list of the outcomes (instead of the older problem list) is revolutionary in terms of turning thinking, planning, and documenting from a task-driven to an outcomes-based approach. An excerpt of such a plan of care outcomes list follows.

Figure 18-1   Interdisciplinary Plan of Care

Patient Name: _____

Diagnosis/Procedure: _____

Instructions: All disciplines will document identified patient outcomes and goals.

PLANNED PATIENT OUTCOME	STATUS
Nursing_____ Physician_____ OT/PT_____ Dietary_____ Case Mgmt_____ Resp_____	Met ☐
	Date/Signature _____
	Revised ☐
	Date/Signature _____

13. **In this hospital, shift report is mostly a review of interventions for each patient, even though they are listed on the MAR (medication administration record) and treatment record. How do I get nurses to give a more outcome-oriented report? They say it is more time-consuming that way, and many nurses are anxious to get out on time and not have to wait for the new shift to finish report.**

> First of all, it is important to understand that report serves many purposes, beyond the obvious need to communicate plans and to hand off care to the next team. There is a social context to report as well, and many nurses use this time to connect to colleagues, to share stories, and to validate the work they do. This type of social interaction may be time-consuming, but is seen as an essential cultural component of who we are and how we see each other.

> By far, the best report is a face-to-face exchange from colleague to colleague, in front of the patient. However, the reluctance to do this form of sharing is typically monumental, and nurses seek to find ways to retreat to the quiet safety of the lounge or the station, or the office, where they can review the care more privately. With the patient out of the picture, is it possible to really think and plan critically for the ongoing consistent care the patient needs?

> If a face-to-face, "walking rounds" approach is met with too much resistance, try facilitating outcomes discussions and critical exchange using Figure 18-2. This way of categorizing the data is based on work by William Bridges in his leading change books and is exceptionally useful in many applications. The "four Ps" are part of Bridge's suggested way of handling transition, and I have added clarifiers specific to what the nurses of a particular surgical unit wanted to hear during report. This facilitates their ownership in the process, and creates more success.

14. **Nurses are an aging workforce. Are there specific considerations for the nurse who is now well over 40?**

> I think it is essential that we analyze the workforce, consider the special needs and focus of each work group, and work together for creative approaches and solutions. How does the new young graduate fit in with a team of nurses over the age of 50 who are both experienced and have been in the same area for many years? There is a distinct difference in their attitudes, values, and concerns. We need to challenge the assumptions we are making, look for specific validated differences, and begin to address those, rather than conjecturing that we will continue to "eat our young."

PURPOSE: To share information about the patients, in order for the plan of care to be continuous and effective, based on the patients' desired outcomes.

PICTURE: Create a clinical picture of the patient by including the following:

- Patient name, room number, age, physician (who is covering), and diagnosis
- Date of surgery, post-op day
- Code status
- Pertinent past history
- I/O, weight, vital signs and blood sugars: how often done, if there are any changes such as fever, weight gain or loss, hyper/hypotension, hyper/hypoglycemia
- Any changes in condition that are not within the expected clinical path for the patient

PLAN: Identify what is being supported in terms of patient outcomes and problems

- Pain management: PCA, last medication and effectiveness
- Fluid management: IVs, rate, and condition of site
- Activity: assistance and progress
- Diet: type, whether tolerating and progressing
- Elimination: catheter, voiding, assistance, bowel program
- Procedures: surgery, lab work, diagnostics, and time scheduled, prep needed
- Respiratory status: use of oxygen, lung sounds, effort, chest tubes
- Wound/dressing: status and who changes/when
- Education: for family and/or patient regarding management of diagnosis
- Discharge plans: estimated date of discharge and where going, who is helping, what is necessary to prepare

PART: Identify who has been doing what, for this patient, and who needs to carry on the following shift

- Other disciplines involved—respiratory, dietary, PT, diabetic teaching
- Specifics the UAP needs to pay attention to: fluid restriction, safety issues, restraints, frequent monitoring
- Permits, orders, and plans the licensed staff needs to complete
- Coordination of care that the RN needs to continue to support what is most important for the patient in terms of goals this shift

Figure 18-2: Shift Report

A recent study resolved to focus on retention of older nurses. A researcher (Susan Letvak at UNC Greensboro) studied 400 RNs ages 45–65 and identified the importance of relationships; their motivation for caring; their need for recognition; that health concerns need not be a barrier (94% indicated that they met most of the physical demands of the job most of the time). This invalidates the assumption that older nurses are worried about the physical demands and challenges us to reconsider the more important issues of recognition and opportunities for caring.

15. How can we best use critical thinking to meet the needs of the staff, keep them happy enough to stay, and excited about the work they do?

Well, that's a book in itself! Seriously, I would start with the question process, as in all critical thinking. What does the staff want? While this is a general inquiry, and much too broad in scope, the challenge is to narrow it to the point where the information you receive is useful. Consider shaping the question as "What is the perfect shift?" This can be the opening for a staff/department meeting or a question you post in the lounge on a flip chart and invite comments. The responses are generally very telling, and will indicate if there is an emphasis and focus on quality of work life issues (e.g., a perfect shift is getting out on time, having time to go to the bathroom, getting a break, having only X number of patients) or an emphasis on quality of patient care (e.g., having time to meet patients' needs, making a difference with someone, being able to assist patients in improving their current status, teaching patients what they need to do to achieve their goals). Too often, managers and leaders use a "shotgun" approach and offer a smattering of recruitment/retention strategies in hopes that some staff will be appreciative. Instead, begin with assessment and validate those assumptions that you may be tempted to act upon before you buy the movie tickets or the free lunch coupons!

16. What can I do on a daily basis to foster critical thinking in staff?

I think that good coaching and leading behaviors are helpful on all levels. If you care enough to spend the time to ask the staff, then by all means, make certain you respond to the suggestions offered! Failure to do so results in frustration, extinguishes enthusiasm, and leads people to the door. To retain staff, and to develop them, consider using the behaviors in Table 18.2. Make them a habitual part of your daily approach, and you will see the positive results!

TABLE 18.2 Coach and Leader Behaviors

- Coaching rather than blaming
- Encouragement of healthy conflict and diverse perspectives
- Questions/risk taking supported
- Challenging frames of reference, attitudes, assumptions
- Modeling of openness, risk taking, clarity, consistency, specificity, willingness to take a stand and to change opinion based on evidence
- Establish networks of peer support
- Affirming self-worth; attentive listening

RESOURCES

Kelly Thomas, K. J. (1998). *Clinical and nursing staff development: Current competence, future focus.* Philadelphia: Lippincott.

Kaye, B., & Jordan-Evans, S. (2002). *Love'em or lose'em: Getting good people to stay* (2nd ed.). San Francisco: Berrett-Koehler Publishers, Inc.

Porter-O'Grady, T., & Wilson, C. K. (1995). *The leadership revolution in health care: Altering systems, changing behaviors.* Gaithersburg, MD: Aspen.

Appendix:
The Elephant Dances with Creative Ideas!

Here the contributors share some of their creative approaches.

1. **Stimulation**
   Elizabeth E. Hand, MS, RN, CCRN

2. **Great Activities**
   Bette Case, PhD, RN, BC

3. **More Ideas**
   Rozalinda Alfaro-LeFevre, MSN, RN

4. **More Options**
   Marilynn Jackson, PhD, MA, RN

1. Stimulation

One of the critical thinking exercises I use with novice critical care nurses to stimulate their thinking relates to identifying ways to indirectly measure cardiac output/cardiac index (whether the patient has or does not have a Swan-ganz catheter in place). If they need some priming, I tell them to watch the UOP and that usually gets a discussion going. I e-mailed that comment to a colleague and received some of the funniest suggestions about what UOP could stand for—Unidentified Organizational Personnel? So now, if the lecture needs some stimulation or humor, I ask people what else UOP could stand for (it stands for urine output) and after some laughter we all feel refreshed.

2. Great Activities

Turn-the-Question-Around

This is something I do that makes active learning of one of the points made in the book—that sometimes nurses or leaders are too quick to give a definitive answer. Sometimes reflecting the question, rephrasing the question, or probing with a question will stimulate critical thinking on the part of the person who raised the question initially. This also helps the person who was asked the question to clarify what it is that the person who asked is *really* asking.

Ask participants to form pairs. Then ask each individual, as an individual, to think of some question that he/she is frequently asked. (For faculty it's often "What's going to be on the test?"; for nurse managers and other leaders it's often "When are we getting more staff?") Then direct the partners to take turns—first one asks the other the question. Then the partner who has been asked asks as many questions as he/she can think of to clarify or lead the questioner to answers. The rule is that the questions must not require simple yes or no responses.

This requires a demonstration by the presenter—perhaps on one of the questions given as examples above—for "What's on the test?" it would be "Where would that fit in the test plan I gave you?" or, "How does that fit with the course objectives?" or, "If you were writing the test what kind of a question would you ask?" For the staffing question, "What would another staff member be doing?" "What other ways can we organize the assignments?" "Who else could help?" or "If we could have someone perform some of the care needed by patients, what would those aspects be?"

This exercise can be fun if at least the presenter and perhaps a few others wear the beanie hats with the spinners on top. When the presenter first demonstrates, he/she can say *turn-the-question* around and spin the spinner. When the presenter asks for a few of the pairs to report on their questioning, the pair reporting can wear the beanies.

Crush the Butterfly

This exercise illustrates the need for structure and freedom to co-exist. This is really a metaphor for research methods—that they need to be rigorous enough to capture the phenomenon, but not so heavy-handed as to destroy the phenomenon they mean to describe. For this exercise, I make a paper butterfly. The butterfly may represent critical thinking among staff or for an individual student, or it may represent quality care or other concepts of interest.

I let the butterfly rest in my hand, palm up with my fingers spread and flexed slightly to contain the butterfly. Then relax the fingers and with the other hand let the butterfly "fly away" with the description that fits the concept. Return the butterfly to the original position in the palm, gently contained by the fingers. Then describe heavy-handed tactics that fit the concept and close the hand to a fist to crush the butterfly.

The CT Introduction

I demonstrate this first myself. I ask participants to list their three initials in a vertical format. (It's always fun to give anyone who has no middle initial the choice of any of the 26 letters.)

Then I direct them to let the first initial represent something they want to get out of the session; the second initial to represent a challenge of theirs; the last initial to represent a great strength, or if they're feeling modest, something for which they receive compliments and kudos. The initial can be used as the first letter of the response, or incorporated.

After a minute, I ask them to share their compositions with those at their table, or another colleague.

Before debriefing, I ask if anyone had trouble coming up with a strength that begins with or incorporates their last initial. If anyone comes forward, I ask the group to give him/her suggestions (works best of course if there are others in the group who know the person). That suggests a nice affirming variation on this technique (instead of asking participants to identify their own strengths, you can just ask the group or another person to respond).

I debrief this as an illustration of the left-brain and right-brain sides of critical thinking. The left-brain is represented by the initials which are the givens, even though they may have changed over time *and* by the arbitrary concepts I told them to represent. This represents the context and givens within which critical thinking as nurses occurs (e.g., principles of pathophysiology, pharmacology, policies and procedures). However, the responses they came up with were generated, unique, creative responses *to fit the criteria*. The activity also illustrates the many-right-answers nature of critical thinking.

Acronym Summary

Similar to the above, I sometimes close by laying out C-R-I-. . . (critical thinking) vertically and asking the group to shout out concepts or characteristics that relate to CT. It's also fun to advise groups of educators that if they do this with the topic of the day, they have to be prepared to hear what the group got out of the session compared with what they intended (how it comes out vs. the intended outcome).

Multiple-Choice Introduction

This is a simple matter of asking participants to create an multiple choice question of the form "Which of the following is *not* true about me?" for which they create choices that are three true statements and untrue statement. They then try the question out on participants with whom they are seated. It's fun, a good ice breaker, and can be debriefed in a variety of ways including highlighting perspectives and assumptions. In test construction workshops I use it to point out principles of multiple choice construction, including why negatively stated stems are inadvisable and that common misunderstandings make the best distracters.

A variation is to create a multiple choice assignment that is conceptually linked to the content. For example in "Change" sessions, I have asked participants to create a multiple-choice question, "Which of the following changes have I experienced in my life?" This has rich possibilities for encouraging sharing about characteristics of change—loss, grief, acceptance, gains, who gains and what is gained.

Another variation for sessions on adult learning and developing teaching techniques is, "The most effective way for me to learn is . . . "

Obviously these can be short-answer questions but the multiple choice format is a little more fun.

Modified Version of the Six Hats

Depending upon the size of the group, there are numerous ways to create groups which will present the assigned perspective on an issue. The issue may be one which the whole group identifies, or it may be one that the presenter supplies.

I sometimes make nurses' caps out of colored paper—although nurses' caps are a dated concept, it makes another point about perspectives (e.g., our predecessors in nursing, different times, cultures).

The White Hat

Information: Think white paper

What information do we need?

What does that information tell us?

The Yellow Hat

Optimism: Think sunshine

What are the positives about visitors in the unit?

What fantastic outcomes can we obtain this way?

The Black Hat

Pessimism: Think storm cloud

What are the negatives about visitors in the unit?

What terrible things will happen if we change our policy?

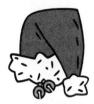

The Red Hat

Feelings: Think valentine heart

Whose feelings do we need to consider?

What exactly are the feelings of those parties?

The Green Hat

Creativity: Think growing green plant

What wild and crazy ideas can make this work?

What else?

The Blue Hat

Clarification/Direction: Think clear blue sky or pilot

What needs clarification?

What perspective has not been heard from?

Note: From deBono, E. (1985). *Six thinking hats*. Larchmont, NY: The International Center for Creative Thinking.

In large groups, I arrange for each person to choose a colored paper badge, colored pen, or other item that corresponds to one of the perspectives. I place a mix at each table as groups are seated. I then designate meeting places for each perspective with table signs. Then, those seated at the table come up with their assigned perspective and report it to the group.

In smaller groups, pairs or groups of 3–4 can be assigned to each perspective and write the points of their perspective on flip charts posted around the room. It's fun to give them hats to wear. I usually retain the blue hat for myself as director, moderator, and clarifier of the discussion.

For whatever method you choose to allow groups to outline their perspectives, the final step is a discussion in which all engage after reporting the points they have identified within each perspective.

3. More Ideas

I believe in what I call the WLI Approach (give them something to wonder, laugh, and interact about) within the first 10 minutes. They may all be different things, but it happens within the first 10 minutes. One thing I do is put a funny-looking "Devil's Advocate" card up on the overhead and tell participants that they're invited to play the "Devil's Advocate" card at anytime because when objections are raised, we all learn more. I also put up a "Survivor Card" on the overhead and tell them at the end of the program, they'll vote for the person in the room who, based on the person's willingness to contribute to the group, they would best like to have with them if they were stuck on a workplace island. That person gets a prize. It's interesting to me that *every time*, the person who gets voted the Survivor has been the person who has been most verbal with difficult questions. It takes courage to ask difficult questions. And, it has also has raised my level of ability to respond to difficult questions!

4. More Options

Emotional Connections

To connect emotions and logic, I have participants think about the three most significant decisions they have made so far in their lives. I then ask them to consider whether the decisions were based primarily on logic or emotion, and why. This always inspires great discussion and eye-opening awareness of the connections between emotion and logic.

Warm-Ups and Jokes

I also love to use jokes, and have found the listserv of **listmom@strive.to** a great place to subscribe to daily humor.

The Black Dot

At the start of a meeting, I like to draw a large black dot in the middle of a flip chart and then ask participants to describe what they see. It is always interesting to hear the variety of answers, and they will almost always focus on the black dot, describing it literally (a misshaped circle in the middle of the page) to creatively (the black eye of a white rabbit in a snowstorm). The message is, of course, to get them to see outside of the black dot, to focus on the surrounding white, and to state that critical thinking is about seeing the whole picture, not just one narrow spot on the page.

Professional Stereotyping

In order to help participants to get in touch with the source of some of their assumptions, I have used a tool that challenges staff to identify what they think about certain professions. To help dispel age-old attitudes, use the following categories in a handout, or as the basis of a discussion in a staff meeting:

	What I think about	**Where I got that image**
Motorcycle rider	Black leather, Hell's angel, trouble, gangs	Movies, bad experience when growing up
Physical therapist		
Physician		
Social worker, etc...		

Five Minute Think

This is also known as "sitting with the question" and comes from a number of sources. Michelangelo used it, as does Edward de Bono—both suggesting that we do not spend enough time in careful consideration of the question itself, and are in too much of a hurry to reach a resolution. When you pose a problem or a question, invite the staff or the participants to take a few minutes (time them) to sit quietly with the issue, and to consider what the question really is asking. This is tough to do, and I have found that sometimes I just need to have the group sit for 30 seconds to see what that amount of time is really like. This answers the rebuttal, "We don't have enough time to think!"

Board Games

We have talked about the need to exercise the brain, to stimulate thought, and to keep us growing in the most positive ways. There are several board games that help do that, and I have found that just taking a piece of the game to start a staff meeting, or at a staff lunch, or to begin a shift report, helps get everyone thinking and "warmed up."

Place *Trivial Pursuit* cards in the staff lounge, or have a few at the desk or in the nurses' station. You can do the same thing with the cards from *Mind Trap*, another wonderful game with a deck of cards that have interesting questions on them, all designed to make you think.

Cranium is another great game for exercising both sides of the brain, as is *Scrabble*. I am sure that you can think of many more—be creative and have fun!

Index